The Back Pain Bible

A Breakthrough Step-By-Step Self-Treatment Process
To End Chronic Back Pain.

Copyright

Publisher: Influential Health Solutions LLC

Lighthouse Point, Florida, U.S.A.

Published June, 29th 2017

ISBN-13: 978-0998590653

DISCLAIMER:

Neither the author nor the publisher assumes any responsibility for errors, omissions, or contrary interpretations of the subject matter herein. Any perceived slight of any individual or organization is purely unintentional.

Cover Design: Christopher J. Kidawski

Author's photo courtesy of: Christopher Haugh

Also By Chris

The Death Of Dieting: Lose Weight, Banish Allergies, and Feed Your Body What It Needs To Thrive!

The Everspace: Utilizing the Power Of God and Neuroscience To Create Stillness Within.

The Ultimate Self-Help Guide For Joint Pains: Back, Head, Neck, Shoulder, Knee, Foot & Ankle.

The Knee Pain Bible: A Self-Care Guide to Eliminating Knee Pain and Returning to The Movements You Love!

The Foot & Ankle Pain Bible: A Self-Care Guide to Eliminating The Source of Your Foot Pain.

The Head, Neck & Shoulder Pain Bible: A Self-Care Guide to Eliminating Upper Body Pain.

Not Your Average Paleo Diet Cookbook: 100 Delicious & Healthy (Mostly) Lectin-Free Recipes!

Not Your Average Vegan Instant Pot Cookbook: 100 Delicious & Healthy Recipes!

Not Your Average Paleo Cookbook: 100 Delicious & Healthy (Mostly) Lectin-Free Recipes!

Advanced Praise

“Not only is Chris a gifted athlete and a skilled trainer, in his new book he draws from years of experience of trial and error. He condenses this information to dispel the myths surrounding back injury, and helps you get to the root of your problem quite easily. The book gives us a clear understanding of the importance of self-care through regular, consistent mobility work. It is a must-read for elite athletes, beginners, and individuals of all body types.”

Jeff Oppenheimer, MD
Neurosurgeon

“I can not even explain how grateful I am for what Chris has done; this book is a true miracle worker! If it wasn't for him, I'd be stuck with my old problems and for the past few years I could feel something was wrong with my body, yet nobody could help me. After utilizing the techniques in this book I immediately found that my glutes were locked up and not firing correctly. Since utilizing his mobility sessions I have drastically reduced pain in my back and I finally feel like I'm on the right path!”

Malin S.

"Chris Kidawski has helped me to stay injury free my entire football career. His techniques have helped me recover from sprained ankles, muscular trauma, and a broken back in record time. The guidance he provides in this book to me is invaluable."

Davone Bess
Former NFL Wide Receiver

Dedication

This book is dedicated to all those in pain who have been searching for a way to move freely again.

Table of Contents

Copyright 2

Dedication 7

Foreword 11

Your Back Pain: Friend or Foe? 13
My Story: It Wasn't About the Pain 15

Chapter 1 – You Are Not a Robot 19
The Fascial Network 21
Your Body Is a Closed Loop 22
The Problem vs. The Symptom 24
Ask the Coach: Why Has Nothing Helped In the Past? 27

Chapter 2 – Move More Aware 30
What Happens Between 4 and 44? 32
Practice Makes Permanent 36
Your Body Is a Yes Man 37
The Word of the Day: Pressure 39
Ask the Coach: Can I Exercise Through All of This? 41

Chapter 3 - Is It Mobility or Motility? 44
Are You Cool Like That? 45
3 Keys to Success 47
The Kaizen Principle 50
How Long Will This Take? 51
Ask the Coach: What Makes This Different from Other Approaches? 52

Chapter 4 - An Intricate Marriage 54
We Don't Know What We Don't Know 55
Your Feet Tell All 56
Your Sacred Seat: The Hip Flexors 60
Your Abs Are Not Your Core 62
You Don't Have Back Pain, You Have a Butt Problem 63
The Gluteus Minimus 66

The Gluteus Medius....67
The Gluteus Maximus....68
The Hamstrings....70
Bonus: The Deep Muscles of the Pelvis....71
Ask the Coach: What About Icing My Back?....72

Chapter 5 – Step 1: Mobility.... 77
Called to Care....80
Abdominal Mobility....81
Hip Flexor Mobility....87
Gluteus Minimus Mobility....90
Gluteus Medius Mobility....93
Gluteus Maximus Mobility....96
Hamstring Mobility....98
Into the mind of the coach: Knowing your "WHY."....100
Lower Back Mobility....101
Ask The Coach: Sitting or Standing Desk?....106

Chapter 6 – Step 2: Stretching....108
Why We Have to Do It....110
Stretching Rules and Plasticity vs. Elasticity....111
Two Tests....116
The Modified Lunge....119
The Couch Pose Stretch....122
The 75 – 90 – 120 Stretch....125
The Hip Flexor Stretch with Rotation....131
The Van Damme Stretch....138
Your Keys to Success....143
Ask the Coach: Should I Go See a Massage Therapist? 144

Chapter 7 – Step 3: Motility....146
Neuromuscular Reprogramming....148
Strengthening The Back....150
Band Walks....152
Deep Hip Hinge Abduction....158
Banded Good Morning....162
Walking Lunges....166
The Four Way Glute Bridge....172

Bent Knee Single Leg Glute Bridge 178
Concluding Thoughts on Strength 181
Ask the Coach: Why does all of this stuff (rolling, stretching, strengthening) have to hurt? Is that good? 181

Chapter 8 – Troubleshooting 185
Common Struggles 186
Consistency 187
Patience 189
Nutrition 190
Stress Levels 193
Supplements 197
Ask the Coach: How Important Is Sleep? 200

Chapter 9 - Putting It All Together 203
If the Pieces Fit 204
Sample Program 205
My Wish for You 207
Ask the Coach – How Do I Become a Client? 208

You're Giving Back! 214

Foreword

Let me preface the following statement by agreeing with you if it seems that this is just another puff piece that must be too good to be true. Hearing results with a laundry list of superlatives immediately triggers the cynicism in all of us, but for those willing to listen, I am here to tell you in fact that there aren't enough of said superlatives to describe the results I have seen. A high-level athlete who had previously received regular treatments with extremely positive results first referred me to Chris. As mentioned above, I carried with me a high degree of skepticism that my chronic, at times debilitating, back/knee pain had zero chance of being resolved due in large part to many failed attempts with physical therapy in the past. Despite short-term success with frequent and pricey physical therapy visits the results were never permanent, resulting in increased frustration and decreased physical activity.

Chris' myofascial release techniques coupled with what can be described as biomechanical reprogramming combine for a treatment modality that is less invasive than injections or surgery, while also providing better long-term results than even the most aggressive physical therapy plans. Having experienced the aforementioned never-ending paradox of orthopedic surgeon consults and physical therapy treatment plans myself, I can say (happily) that not only have these methods allowed me to continue to participate pain free in a variety of athletic activities, but also have given me the tools to maintain said results with minimal effort.

Fully believing that my results were not an outlier I have also advised colleagues of mine to see Chris, with all experiencing similarly positive outcomes. To anyone out there using chronic pain as a crutch for not being active, I would challenge them to give what you will find in this book a chance prior to undergoing painful injections or unnecessary surgical procedures.

Chad A. Boatman D.O
PGY-1 Emergency Medicine

Your Back Pain: Friend or Foe?

"Lack of activity destroys the good condition of every human being, while movement and methodical physical exercise save it and preserve it." –Plato

Before you start reading, I'd like you to do an exercise for me. Get somewhere quiet, sit as comfortably as you can, and set a timer for one minute. Close your eyes and pay attention to your breath. Feel your heart beat. Feel your toes, maybe they're cold, maybe you can feel their strength and all they do for you each day. Feel your blood running through your veins utilizing every effort it can to keep you alive and healthy. When the timer goes off, open your eyes and then come back to where you left off.

Did you do it? I really hope so. The reason for having you do that exercise is because I want you to realize your body is your friend. *Time* is your friend! In those 60 seconds alone your body went through 6 billion chemical reactions (it has been studied we produce 100 million chemical reactions per second while resting). I know you're in pain. I know you may feel like you're sleeping with the enemy, or as if you are wasting your days away not being able to live as fully as you are used to. This pain you're experiencing is not happening *to* you, it is happening *for* you! Pain is an indicator we are still alive. Pain is a reminder for me of how fragile life can be and to never take a moment for granted. In order for you to heal yourself fully, you need to change the way your brain thinks about pain.

Now that we got that out of the way, I want to share with you some good news. You are holding in your hands a refined, step-by-step approach I use to eliminating more than 99% of the low back pain cases I deal with. The only people I have not been able to help have had fractures in their spine, which only time is able to heal. The approach I am going to reveal to you has helped cure or manage back pain resulting from:

- Herniated, or bulging disks
- Post back surgery pain
- Slips, falls, or car accidents
- Weightlifting/sport-related trauma

Please do not panic if you don't see the cause of your back pain in the above bullets. The approach we will be taking is both universal as well as individual. You may have to work harder in one modality and not so much in another, where someone else may have to work in the complete opposite fashion to achieve optimal results. The bottom line here is we are all different, but the same. It's not how we got hurt, but how we heal that makes the process different or individual.

Best-selling author Vishen Lakhiani states that 95% of the population is still stuck in a victim mentality.

Not you. By buying this book, you can no longer consider yourself to be helpless. The people I learn from, and myself included all say the same thing – *you are your own best therapist.* Until some forward-thinking company builds a machine that allows me to feel what you feel, the application of these methods is up to you. Realize too that you are one of many. There have been hundreds of others whom I helped, who felt lost and hopeless at the beginning and now enjoy their freedom and peace of mind knowing their body is returned to health. Rest assured I will apply the same dogged determination in your case as I did in theirs. Many blessings to you on your journey!

My Story: It Wasn't About the Pain

I can't remember a single time when I was younger where I wasn't moving. From a very young age I was already playing five different sports: golf, hockey, baseball, basketball, and football. Not that an 8-year-old child knows anything about sanity, but moving kept me sane. There were times I remember being locked inside all day due to a terrible snow storm and as I would try to fall asleep my legs would still be going and I would end up tossing and turning all night. I would spaz out from time to time having uncontrollable energy and my mother would tell others I had "episodes" – whatever that meant. As my time as a collegiate athlete came to a close, it was no wonder I couldn't accept sitting behind a desk as an actual job. Rather than become a professional athlete, I figured training people to become professional athletes would be a great path in life to take and my intuition served me well.

I started training athletes at The University at Buffalo (UB) in August of 1999, even before I had my Certified Strength and Conditioning Specialist certification. My enthusiasm about lifting weights, running faster, and jumping higher was shining through to every group I coached and I soon started to make a name for myself as the guy you wanted to see to improve performance. I was devouring books, signing up for more certifications, and listening to what cues my superiors used to communicate effectively with their athletes. I didn't feel like I was at work and I liked that, but the hyper-rewarding feeling I got from seeing someone improve at their craft became addicting and I realized that while I was in this profession to make money, and ultimately a living, the true benefit was the people I was helping.

About a year into my stint at UB, I was performing a power clean exercise where I take the bar from the ground and lift it up to my shoulders in one smooth motion. As I was lifting the bar on my fifth and final rep, I jumped my feet out as I did hundreds of times before to put my body in a good position to receive the bar and my left foot landed in a puddle of my sweat shooting my foot left, and causing my knee to cave in. Being young and full of testosterone, I was determined to save the lift and as I strained to recover there was a quiet little pop that echoed from the left side of my lower back. I stood up with the bar, dropped the weight and triumphantly walked over to the water fountain, victorious. My victory was short lived, however.

As I bent over to take a drink of water, my back completely gave out on me and I had to suspend myself on the fountain with my arms or risk head butting a sheet of steel. Then the pain appeared. It felt like someone had secured a pickaxe and driven it through my lower lumbar while I was taking my sip of water. This created a spasm in my diaphragm which rendered taking a deep breath nearly impossible. What was happening to me? I pushed myself away from the fountain and walked back into the weight room, calmly removed the weights from my bar (which gave me that neat little pickaxe feeling I mentioned earlier every time I bent over) and walked over to see the athletic trainers.

The frustration that ensued for nearly 2.5 months while I tried to heal my back was shocking, to say the least. I entrusted myself to the care of nearly 5 different practitioners whom each had their slew of gizmos and gadgets for assessing what was wrong with my back. After every appointment I was met with the same response: "We just don't know." MRIs were showing nothing, X-rays were showing nothing, and muscle sensation tests showed I had full feeling and proprioception in all of my extremities. Not a single doctor could find out what was wrong with me or why the pain was so persistent. Walking hurt, sitting hurt, laughing, coughing, and sneezing were excruciating. With as much discomfort as I was in, there was one solid conclusion my frustration was leading to and that was *it wasn't about the pain!*

Being an athlete, pain was a constant part of my life. What I was not used to was the same pain lingering for months on end that was actually inhibiting me from doing what I loved. Even though I could move, I felt paralyzed. Movement for me used to be unconscious, automatic, and taken for granted! Now I had to think about my every step. If I dropped my keys, I would have to plan the least painful route for picking them up. Ask anyone who has had any form of back pain and they will concur: it's with you 24/7. While all of this was concerning me on a day-to-day basis, my greatest frustration was why the people who are supposed to be able to help me, were not able to help me! I felt lost, and often worried if I would ever be the same again. Was I going to need surgery? Was my career as a strength and conditioning coach over before it even began? Not only was the pain knotting up my back, but also the uncertainty of all of this was knotting up my stomach. At wits' end, I took to playing WEB MD and decided I was going to have to fix myself.

I researched tirelessly and what I found was that I was not alone. There were tens of thousands of people out there on the Internet in pain forums looking for the same answers I was. Unfortunately, the answers being presented by people trying to help were less than ideal. Popping pills, taking shots, or having surgery was not an option for me especially with surgery having a whopping 30% cure rate. Physical therapy wasn't showing any promise either, as most people were reporting a minimal decrease in pain at best. To beat this I realized I was going to have to innovate, and innovate I did.

Chapter 1 – You Are Not a Robot

"The fascia is the place to look for the causes of diseases and the place to begin treatment." –A.T. Still Philosophy of Osteopathy, 1899

Manny is not your average real estate agent. In his early 20s, he served in the army with distinction and had become accustomed to the grind and physical-ness that the military ingrains in all of its participants. Now in his early 50s, you can still find him kayaking with his family, climbing the random tree just for fun, and playing basketball with his children and their friends. He notices that the longer the drive when hunting for a great home, the longer it takes him to loosen up when he gets out of his car. He chalks it up to old age and goes back to focusing on his business. Soon after that, Manny notices that not only is his back tight after his long rides, but he is also getting a pain shooting from the left side of his back down into his leg. This really has his attention now, as the pain seems to worsen week-to-week. He goes to see his primary care physician and is prescribed muscle relaxers but those don't help him any. He goes to the chiropractor and even though there are a few cracks and pops, the pain is still there when he wakes up the next day. After talking with a friend one day he hears about me, and calls to make an appointment.

Our very first session together I give him a range of motion test and find his left Gluteus Maximus (butt muscle) to be much tighter than his right. I ask him if he can remember any injury he had that would cause such an imbalance between the two sides of his body and as he paused to think about it I suddenly saw his eyes light up. About four years ago he was playing with his children by the pool and slipped on the deck. As he landed on his right butt cheek pretty hard, he also extended his right arm to break his fall. Thinking he was still a young buck in the army he laughed it off and went about playing with his children. He remembered that his right hip was sore for about two weeks after the fall!

This type of case happens more often than you would think. The trauma caused to the muscle and its fascia from the fall was never attended to. Manny's brain then unconsciously started to favor his right leg and overcompensate with his left, which caused the muscle surrounding that hip to tighten and compress nerves sending the pain down his leg. This specific type of pain is called "referred" pain and is what keeps practitioners chasing their tails with tough cases they can not figure out how to heal. The practitioner is treating the symptoms rather than the problem, and the reason this doesn't work is because *we are not robots!*

The Fascial Network

Allow me to confuse you for one second. Human beings are machines, but we are not robots. When I see someone walking in for his or her first appointment, I see a machine, not a human. I see levers, I see angles, I look to see where their feet are facing, and whether or not their hips are level. You don't have to be a mechanic to know something is wrong with your engine if a pungent black smoke is pouring out of it, right? When we do take our car to the mechanic all he does is swap out parts. He says this is broken, so I gave your car a new one. The human body, however, does not work this way in most cases. In most cases if your back is broken, you have a butt problem. Your butt problem will also cause a hamstring problem, which does not allow your calf or foot to function correctly.

What we need to understand first and foremost about pain in our body is that it is a lagging indicator of a problem we have had for quite some time now. Most of us think pain is just the beginning when it is in fact the middle of our journey. If your engine seizes up, it didn't just run out of oil that second; it's safe to say the oil was low for a week, maybe two. Pain takes time to develop in our body and some muscles are more resilient to pain than others. Pain travels in the human body because our muscular system is a web. If you pull on a spider web the rest of the web distorts in the direction of that pull until something finally breaks. I care deeply for everyone I help and you are no different. There is a huge mental component to pain and that is why I educate everyone in the same manner. The more we understand, the more we can feel. Feel where our hotspots are. Feel where we are tight. And most importantly, feel what we need to do to become better!

Your Body Is a Closed Loop

I would like you to do an exercise for me right now. Sit comfortably in a chair. Feet on the floor and head held up high. Take three deep breaths and with every inhalation feel where you are tight. Are the aspects of your body responsible for expanding and contracting doing their job? Is there restriction in the belly? Stress in the shoulders? Tightness in the back? It's more than likely you felt one of those three. This is because a web-like structure called fascia surrounds our muscle tissue. In 2001, Thomas Myers wrote a book called *Anatomy Trains* describing how the body is connected from head to toe, and core to cuff. In it he states, "The fascial web so permeates the body as to be part of the immediate environment of every cell." Yes ladies and gentleman, even the backs of our eyes contain fascia, which could be pulling on the back of your neck! Fascia used to be treated as dumb tissue, and largely discarded in anatomy class, but new evidence is showing it to be highly intelligent and one of the prime movers of locomotion and a major friend in our battle against gravity.

To picture fascia, think about it like another skin for our muscles and for our organs. Rather than it separating the outer environment from the inner as our epidermis does, the fascia holds our muscles taut, helps them move with fluidity, and also connects them with information from our organs. We have known muscles are tied to our organs for years now. If your appendix bursts, your abdominal wall turns to a sheet of steel. If you have kidney stones, your back will ache badly. An indicator of an impending heart attack brings pain into our left shoulder, and so on. Eugen Sandow said back in the late 1800s, "You can't have healthy muscles without first having healthy organs and glands."

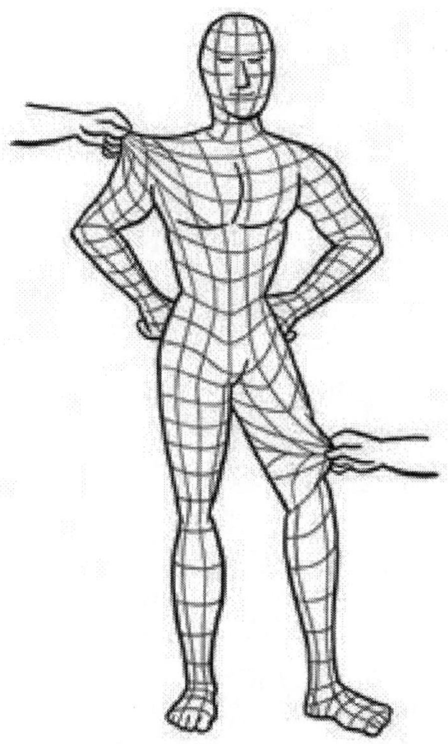

Meet fascia man: Everything is connected – when you pull on the knee, the muscles of the thigh and groin move with it.

The composition of fascia gives us an even clearer picture of why we must be so aware of it. Besides being 65-70% water, fascia is composed of:

Fibroblasts – which give it its shape.
Mastocytes – which aid the immune system and helps secrete hormones.
Adipocytes – fat cells, which reserve energy, and cushion our organs.
Macrophages – which regulate inflammation.
Plasmacytes – which help the immune system organize the defense of the body.
Leukocytes – white blood cells that defend against infection.

Because of its composition, fascia links everything in your body together into one harmonious system. It is in fact a *closed loop, which means it operates based off of feedback from within, and from without of the system*. This is why when we damage a certain area of our body through a fall, a car accident, or sporting injury the pain can spread to other areas of your body.

The Problem vs. The Symptom

Most, if not all of Westernized medicine focuses on treating symptoms, rather than finding and curing the actual problem. Heart disease is treated with pills and open-heart surgery, rather than adjusting the diet. Joint pain is corrected with shots, rather than correcting the way that person is moving. In 2007, $30.3 billion was spent on low back pain. I also indicated that low back surgeries fail over 70% of the time. Today, that number has grown to over $50 billion a year, not to mention the $300-400 billion that is being spent on pharmaceuticals! When it comes to healing the low back, there are several factors we need to be aware of, as we are not just physical beings. Humans are mental, emotional, and spiritual beings, and all of these can factor into back pain. Understanding this, here are some psycho-physiological aspects we need to improve in our life to eradicate and keep back pain away:

Hydration – Stop drinking plastic water! Get a reverse osmosis, Kagan, or AquaTru water filter and always drink from a glass, not a plastic cup. Ditch the 24 packs of water from Costco for $3. The quality of the water matters and there are no testing requirements for bottled water. Being dehydrated will cause your vertebral disks to lose water and compress nerves. Re-hydration usually takes about 90 days.

Your Thoughts – Humans think 80,000 thoughts per day. Research shows over 80% of those are negative. This is psychological weight that tenses us up and compresses the body. It can feel as if real weight is on your shoulders! The best way to eradicate negative thoughts is by starting a meditation practice. Even 10-15 minutes a day can cause a drastic reduction in negative thought production. I reveal in my book The Everspace how neurons that fire together wire together. The more negative thoughts you have, the more predominantly those neurons want to fire. You could be taking a stroll through the park on a beautiful day and then all of a sudden you're trapped in a negative thought pattern of something that happened two years ago for no reason at all. Meditation can be done sitting, or lying – comfort is key. If your mind is running – let it, and soon it will calm itself. A muddy puddle clears up by not disturbing it.

Your Breath – Breathing is the most important function our body performs. You can survive weeks without food or water, but only a few minutes without breathing. When our breathing rates are too high, or the pattern is faulty, the lumbar spine will compensate and pain will develop. Studies show 80% of people using PCs get so engrossed with their work they literally forget to breathe. One doctor has termed this E-mail Apnea. I teach all of my clients to box breathe when working out fascia, but breathing this way throughout the day allows us to remain calmer and control our stress levels because box breathing stimulates the parasympathetic nervous system which is responsible for resting and digesting. To box breathe is simple – inhale through your nose and let your stomach expand for 4 seconds, then exhale through your nose and let your stomach retract for 4 seconds. Breathing this way can do wonders not only for your body, but your mind as well. Start being conscious of your breath today!

Posture – As computers and smartphones control more and more of our lives we find ourselves sitting in terrible chairs, or looking down for too long a period of time and develop conditions like "Text neck." A forward head posture spells disaster for the rest of the spine! Proper posture yields a "Stacked" or neutral spine. We accomplish this by having our shoulders slightly back with our chin slightly tucked whether sitting or standing.

Diet – Eat unhealthy, and your body will be unhealthy. Per my book *The Death of Dieting,* I recommend ditching all processed food. Stick to what nature gave us and you'll be fine, no matter how much of it you eat.

All of the points I just mentioned previously can be problems that eventually contribute to your symptoms. None of them requires you to take a pill, or have surgery to correct. What it does ask you to do is be more mindful of how you operate on a day-to-day basis. As Americans, we love proclaiming how busy we are. We also want what we want fast, and we want it now. At what cost are we willing to live like this? It would be nice to have a private jet, sure, but I don't want someone to have to cart me there in a wheelchair. Correcting back pain as I have illustrated quite extensively in this chapter involves a lot of factors. Your patience is going to be tested many, many times. You need to change the way you think about the body as a closed system, you need to change your negative thoughts to positive, focus on your breathing, consume healthier food, and be more mindful of how you move which we will delve into in greater detail in the next chapter!

Ask the Coach: Why Has Nothing Helped In the Past?

Oftentimes when people come to see me, I am the end of the road for them. I hear story after story about their journey – how much money they spent, how many different practitioners they have seen, who has been telling them what, or how much they've read about their condition. Once again what I hear is it's not about the pain. It's, "Why can't anyone cure my pain?" It's the not knowing what's wrong that's killing them. The main reason that nothing has worked for you in the past is because like my situation, you only have part of the answer, so you achieve partial results. The shots help for a couple weeks, physical therapy only takes some of the pain away, or you feel better for a couple days after the chiropractor. What we fail to realize is how complex the spine is. I took a course called spinal fitness when I was studying for my master's degree and learned some amazing things about the spine. First, the spine is the only structure connecting the pelvis to the shoulders. Second, it contains the spinal cord, which is a super highway for messages from your brain to your entire body. Third, it contains 33 bones: 7 cervical (doctors will sometimes refer to C8 which is a nerve root, not a vertebrae), 12 thoracic (which increase in size as according to their number), 5 lumbar (some people can only have four, while other may have six), 5 sacral (of which all become fused together after age 26), and 3-5 coccygeal (depending on if you're a man or a woman). Fourth, the health of the vertebrae depends on the health of the disks, which is dependent on diet, bodyweight, hydration, our posture, our breathing, our thoughts, and whether or not we exercise.

That little bit of education was designed to help you no longer feel helpless. A complex structure like the spine necessitates a complex solution. There is no silver bullet, no quick fix, no one-size-fits-all cure! One in every 10 million things on this planet is a human being; by your very nature you are a miracle. You are unique and so is your situation. My approach is as comprehensive as it comes. Keep reading and we will find a solution together!

Chapter 2 – Move More Aware

"Healing is a matter of time, but it is sometimes also a matter of opportunity."
–Hippocrates

When Tammy came to see me, she was complaining about a pain in her low back and left hamstring. She knew exactly when she hurt it, but wasn't sure why the pain wasn't going away. Tammy was feeling energized one day in front of her kids and wanted to show them how awesome Mom was still and dropped straight into a split after sitting in a chair for an extended period of time. She heard a loud pop at the bottom of the split and there you have it – instant pain. She told me it would get better and then flare up and no matter what she did or who she went to go see the pain was always a reminder of that faithful day. Did I mention Tammy is 50 years young? Yep, you read that correctly.

As soon as we met I noticed her foot position as she walked in. Her feet were straight ahead - looked good to me. Then my eyes gazed up at her hips. Looked good too. Walking seemed normal, she wasn't favoring her left side, so I knew there was something else going on and I would have to do some more investigative work. As we sat down to talk, there it was, but I reserved judgment and waited a little longer. When we stood up after our conversation there it was again, and that's when I stopped her. When Tammy was calling upon her left leg to produce force, she was favoring it – shifting her hips over to her right side - so I asked her if squatting hurt her hamstring and she said not really. It only radiates pain when she is sitting. My guess was that this movement fault had created a weakness where her glute and hamstring muscles cross in her left leg. Dropping into a split with zero warm-up was obviously too much for it to handle. As we started our mobility session I reinforced proper movement to Tammy and told story after story about how we as human beings need to be more aware of our movement. Faulty movement patterns create tight, weak muscles that are resistant to our own movement! Oftentimes we may not even be aware of them until injury occurs.

Tammy's job until our next appointment was to orient her hips correctly every time before sitting and standing. This included getting into and out of bed, her car, and any time she took a seat. When she came back her first comment was about how hard it was to be conscious of her movement *all* of the time! I agreed and told her how frequently people come into my gym and tell me they can't squat because their knees hurt. I then ask them to demonstrate a proper squat and become horrified by what I see. I tell them my knees hurt just watching! I tell people it is never the 25-50 repetitions you do in the gym that hurt you, it's the 99,000 bad repetitions you do outside of the gym! Another fact is that most injuries in the gym occur at lower than 60% of that person's heaviest weight lifted, which means they were taking their movement for granted and not paying attention to their form. I corrected Tammy's hips, and released the death grip her glute had on her hamstring and the pain went away in 3 weeks. In this chapter, we are going to cover common movement faults, what happens in our body as a result, and how we can *move more aware!*

What Happens Between 4 and 44?

It is a consistent fact of life that as we age we lose our ability to move. Or is it? At 70 years of age, Jack Lalanne—handcuffed, shackled, and fighting strong winds and currents—towed 70 boats with 70 people from the Queen's Way Bridge in the Long Beach Harbor to the Queen Mary, which is one and half miles in distance. How did he do this? Didn't anyone tell him that at 70 years of age he should just be content with withering away in some old folks' home? As the "Godfather of modern fitness" Jack was busy moving his whole life, never allowing for tendons to get stiff or joints to get weak. Nobody in their right mind would park their car for 10 years and expect it to start up and run no problem, yet we have people who sit watching TV, sit in traffic, and sit at work for 10 hours a day in the same position for 10 years, then wonder why they can't bend down to tie their shoes anymore. The simple phrase, "If you don't use it you lose it" rings very true when it comes to the human body.

When we are born our muscular system looks somewhat like this:

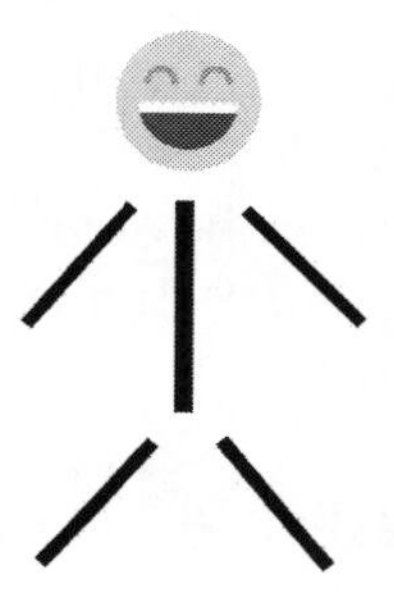

The tissue is soft, healthy and has the ability to expand and contract moving our joints through a full range of motion. After years of prolonged sitting, improper movement, athletic injuries, walking in terrible footwear, and a host of ill-advised lifting techniques learned on YouTube, our muscular and fascial systems start to look like this:

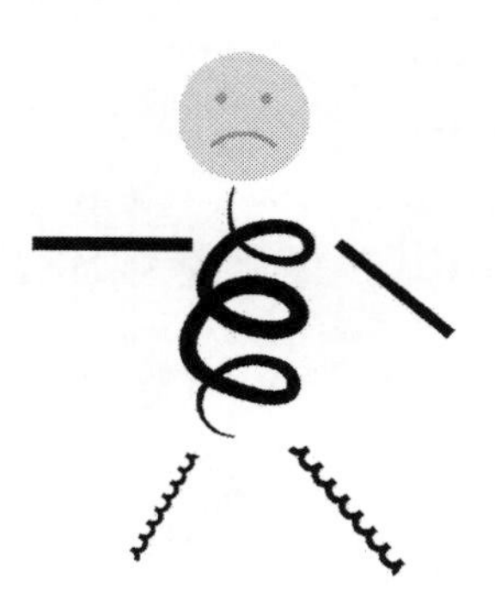

So what happens between the age of 4 and 44? Well that depends on the nature of our movement and what we do with our body. One shoulder may sit higher because we always carry our purse on that side. One leg may be longer from sitting at an angle because it feels more comfortable. And our back and abdominals are a mess from poor posture while sitting, standing, or picking things up with poor form. Another way we can look at this is by illustrating Ida Rolf's block theory of how the body is structured.

This is what we look like when our body is out of sorts:

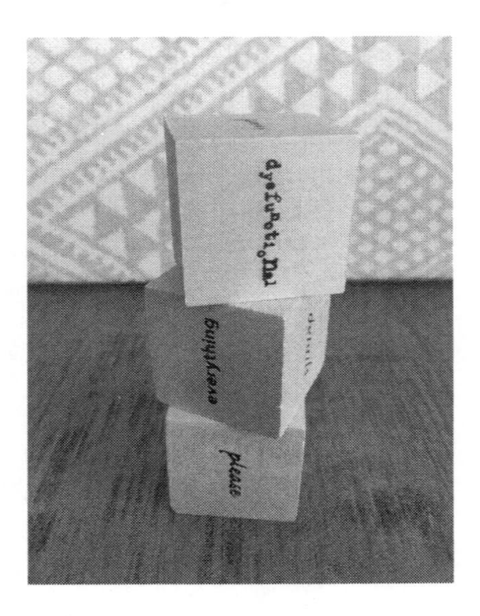

And this is what we want to look like:

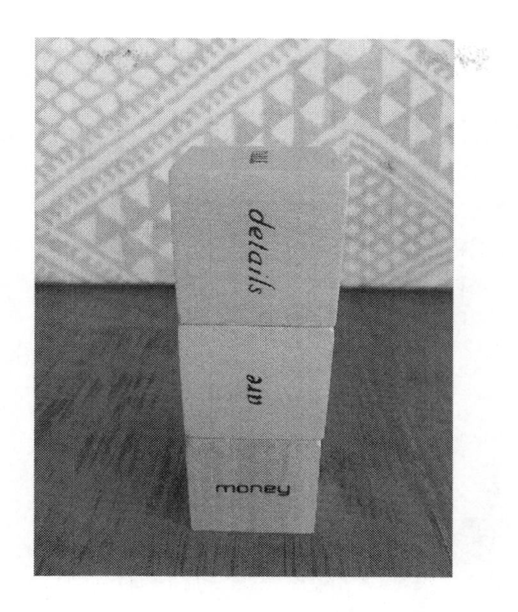

The reason why this occurs as Ms. Rolf so eloquently depicts is because, "In any energy system, however complicated, structure (relationship of units of any size in space) is experienced as behavior." *"Structure is behavior."*

This is basically saying that our body remodels itself according to how we behave. A bricklayer of 40 years will have a terrible back and knees due to the positions he in all honesty "lives" in. In the same respect a baseball pitcher may have an extremely tight throwing arm with some accompanied elbow pain due to how he uses his body in such a repetitive nature. One of the things that can save us here is proper technique, but even technique is not enough in most cases, as we will soon find out.

Practice Makes Permanent

In Daniel Coyle's book *The Talent Code* he talks about how practice does not make perfect in the human body; *it makes things permanent.* Neurons that fire together, wire together in order to make us faster and more efficient at our tasks. In order to understand this more fully, picture someone sitting at a desk.

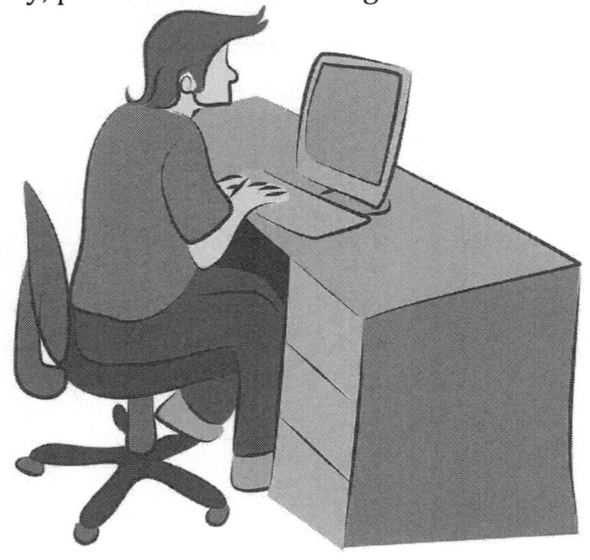

You can see that this person's ankles are at 90 degrees, as well as the knees, and hips. What your body does, when called upon often enough is tighten up the structures of your ankles, knees and hips to produce maximum efficiency in the positions they are mostly in. This means if I need my knees to go a little over my toes, my ankle will have lost the flexibility to do that. What about if I need my butt to go below my knees? You guessed it; you have now lost the flexibility to do that as well. A very easy statement to express this is, "We don't stop playing because we get old; we get old because we stop playing." We are habitual machines and our brain is learning and programming our habits on a second-to-second basis every single day of our lives. When we stop taking our leg through a full range of motion, our brain simply thinks we don't need the full range of motion of that leg anymore thus making the structures tighter. From an evolutionary perspective, why waste the energy if you are not using something? We must remember the body is built for one thing and one thing only and that is survival.

Your Body Is a Yes Man

To illustrate my point and build off of this theory of survival for the human body, here is a pretty shocking story for you. A powerlifter at a gym I used to frequent in Honolulu tore his left pectoral muscle bench pressing and saw it fit to let it heal on its own. His body recovered and even at the age of 49 he could bench press 600 pounds. When he flexed his left chest muscle, you would see it suck right to his sternum, with nothing left attached to the shoulder to stop it. He also had some serious neck and shoulder pain on his left side, and a left tricep that was more developed than his right. The point of telling you this is that when asked, your body will do anything you ask of it, no matter the cost. *Your body is a yes man*! Couple this with the fact that nobody's movement is perfect 100% of the time and this becomes our recipe for pain.

As we move poorly the force we ask our body to develop comes at a cost. We create stressors, or hot spots called trigger points that compress nerves, sending signals back to the brain that there is an injury imminent, or that the muscle tissue is not healthy. The brain then starts to decrease the function of that area which causes the muscles to get weak. When the weakness in the muscle reaches critical limits, the brain sends a new signal to tighten it up in order to protect the joint. Motion in the joint comes at the cost of the motion in the muscle.

Left to germinate for a long enough period of time, pain will soon develop. With all previous warning signs (injury, tightness, weakness) ignored, the trigger points now start to produce pain, but the problem with that is they don't produce pain where they are, they produce pain into the joints those muscles move. We touched on this when we spoke about the problem vs. the symptom. Continuing to move in pain will cause us to compensate our movement in other areas of the body as well, spreading this internal disease. Remember our body is an interconnected web. Putting pressure on any one area is asking the whole body to compensate its movement, not just that specific joint.

An article by Dale G. Alexander, Ph.D. called *Muscle Energy Technique: An Evaluation and Treatment Model for Somatic Dysfunction* states it has been estimated that restriction of one major joint in the lower extremity can increase the energy expenditure of normal walking by as much as 40% and, if two major joints are restricted in the same extremity, by as much as 300%! So let's say you have a tight left hamstring, a muscle we know crosses both the hip and the knee (two joints) in order to properly function. Is it any wonder why your running is getting slower? You are literally asking your body to work 300% harder!!!

If your back is tight is it any wonder why it starts to burn and be uncomfortable while we sit in traffic, or stand in line at the mall for hours on end? The simple fact is tight muscles are unhealthy. They are toxic and sick from not having the space for the capillaries to transport metabolic waste (waste from muscle energy production) away from the muscle, and subsequently transport new nutrients into the muscle to help it recover and grow. To illustrate this further, it would be like walking around with a limited air supply every day. You would limit your movement based off of how much air you had to breathe. The pain sensation you receive from any part of your body is telling you to be careful because time is running out. After reading how our day-to-day movement negatively affects our body, I bet you're wondering what you can do about all of this. The key is simple, yet it's a path not too many are willing to take to get better.

The Word of the Day: Pressure

Pressure, as you know, does some pretty amazing things. It turns peat into coal and coal into diamonds. In the human body, it actually has the reverse effect. It takes little diamonds called trigger points and teaches them to relax, and it takes muscle that is stuck together and helps it glide once again. I tell people time after time that you can always tell how healthy a muscle is by applying pressure. Applying pressure to a muscle should really only refer a pressure sensation back to your brain. If you apply pressure to a muscle and get a pain response back, we now know that muscle is irritated, and has some unhealthy characteristics to it. The by-products of muscle energy production are acidic to the nerves. When musculature becomes tight, it is harder for the circulatory system to get healthy blood into the muscle, and export waste out of the muscle. This creates a toxic environment that can cause atrophy, (decrease in size of the muscle) tightness, and ultimately pain. It is worth noting again to keep at the forefront of our mind that pain is a lagging indicator. It really is the last piece to the puzzle. Most people think pain is just the beginning but it is far from it. Pain is telling you something is breaking or already broken. It's not telling you you have time yet to push yourself. Even though I recommend training through your recovery or recommend using strength movements to garner yourself back to health, we need to realize that we are not smarter than 4 million years of evolution. If we're in pain, we need to slow down.

When we are applying pressure to our muscles we want to make sure we stay in between a pain scale of 6-8, never wandering above that mark. Discomfort is a result of returning our body and its structures to health, but it should never be the purpose. More pressure and more pain do not yield better results. We want to be comfortably uncomfortable. We are not applying pressure to our muscles to achieve a pain scale of 8, working in the 4-6, or 2-4 range is completely acceptable. The reason for this is because when we reach a significant pain threshold, our body fires our sympathetic nervous system, which tells our body to fight against what we are doing. The alarm bells tell our brain to lock up the muscle and since the strength of our muscles is easily greater than any amount of pressure we can apply, by continuing to do so we are wasting our time and energy. You could be using a hammer and chisel and you still will not be able to make a change to the muscle.

One of the key aspects that make my approach unique is making sure we always move when applying pressure to our muscles. The human body heals through movement, not through stabilization, or immobilization. Even something like going for a relaxing barefoot walk in the park or on the beach can calm the central nervous system by grounding ourselves to the magnetism of the Earth, and promote healing. Lying in bed or on the couch for days should be archaic and a thing of the past, but there are still some people that believe rest is the answer.

Now is the time to get excited. We have one more chapter to go through that will define and help us understand this amazing approach that will put your blocks back in order, and return your fascial system to its resting tensegrity. Your pain will soon be a thing of the past!

Ask the Coach: Can I Exercise Through All of This?

This is a question I get all too often. Most people think that because something is hurt, or if we are trying to fix something in the body, that we need as much rest as possible. This is completely false! Like we said in chapter one, your body is a closed loop. This closed loop contains a pump (your heart), a transport system (your blood vessels), and something to be transported (your blood, and its contents). Your blood contains all of the properties necessary to alleviate your pain and restore the elasticity to your muscles, and the plasticity to your fascia. Exercise increases our heart rate and thus increases the amount of healing properties we can get to the recovering area. Sitting on the couch or immobilizing ourselves only ensures we will be in pain for a much longer period of time. Now this doesn't mean that if the lawnmower gets stuck in a ditch we try to rip it out ourselves bursting blood vessels in our eyes. We may want to go get help for that one. When I talk about movement or exercise this can be anything from walking, to rowing, to biking, to training a different body part at the gym. Whatever type of movement does not cause alarming pain—and subsequently increases our heart rate—will do the trick. If you are unable to move or exercise due to your back pain then a sauna or hot tub will do the trick. The simple goal we are trying to achieve is an increase in our heart rate. This speeds up the rate at which our body can get healing properties to the area in question.

All too often, my clients tell me that their previous practitioner advised them to stop everything. In some cases, this added a light case of depression to the worry and anxiety they were feeling due to their pain. I advise all of my clients to continue moving and doing what makes them happy, and find this type of advice speeds up their progress by about 40-50% compared to just resting. Most of the time this is music to my clients' ears because they want to return to as active a lifestyle as possible as soon as possible! As I said earlier, *the human body heals through movement.* Deprive your body of movement and you are encouraging your condition to persist.

Chapter 3 - Is It Mobility or Motility?

"Each patient carries his own doctor inside him."
–Norman Cousins, *"Anatomy of an Illness"*

Mary was an avid weightlifter. She used it as a stress outlet and an avenue to lose weight and feel good. For about 3 years, Mary was progressing very nicely. She had lost close to 30 pounds, was now able to do 15 pull-ups unassisted with just her bodyweight, and deadlifted nearly 225 pounds at a bodyweight of 130 pounds! The deadlift was her most confident exercise so when she saw it in the program for the next day she was excited to show her strength. The workout called for 25 deadlifts at 135 pounds, which was obviously on the lighter side for her. She approached the bar and completed 16 repetitions with no problem at all until she had to rest. She approached the bar again and after pulling two more reps, felt a sharp pain in her low back. She released the bar, consulted her coach and they agreed it was wise for her to bow out of the work out and instead do some mobility for the remainder of class. She drove home and felt fine, only to wake up the next day with horrible back pain.

When Mary came to see me she was confused and concerned. After talking to her for a few minutes and asking her about any previous injuries she told me the only injury she ever had was a broken left leg – just before she started weightlifting. Assessing Mary's flexibility, we found her left glute to be extremely tight. We then assessed her strength on that side and found the glute and the hamstring to be barely firing. I was saddened to tell her that whomever rehabilitated her broken leg had failed to reeducate her glute properly and was in all honestly the main reason why her back gave out. It was like she was picking up the bar with one leg! Utilizing a foam roller, lacrosse ball, a few key stretches and one strength exercise, we restored balance in her hips and eliminated her pain by correcting the problem and not solely working on the symptom.

Are You Cool Like That?

Mobility has been one of those cool buzz words gym goers have been slinging around for a few years now. Synonymous words can also be rolling, foam rolling, smashing, or mobilizing, and are starting to be commonplace in people's warm up and cool down routines. Remember how we just talked about pressure and how it helps take pain away from our muscles? It does this in two ways: First, by sending a signal to the brain to tell the muscles to relax, and second, by draining the energy of these tight angry neurons (single nerve cell). When pressing on adhesions, or trigger points, you can sometimes feel the muscle pulsate or vibrate—this is how you know you have the mobility tool in the right place. By draining the neuron of its energy we get it to give up the constant contraction it is producing which allows the muscle to return to its normal length, decreasing pain and improving its function.

Motility (with a T) is a lesser-known word and because it is literally one letter removed from mobility (with a B) often gets people confused; so let's examine a common case with each.

Let's say Karen has an aching low back for 6 years now. Every move she makes has to be well thought out and calculated because she feels her back can go out at any moment. Whether it's picking keys that she dropped or a long car ride, how her back is going to respond to movement is always at the forefront of her mind. This is a loss of motility (with a T). Motility is commonly referred to in biology in unicellular organisms as the ability to move spontaneously and actively consuming energy in the process. Karen *cannot* move spontaneously and actively due to the pain response in her back. When I talk about motility specifically, I am talking about clearing up entire joints and/or joint processes. Motility is a hostage taker and needs to be dealt with in a different manner pathologically when you are trying to return to health.

Now let's look at Ryan. Ryan is a star short stop for his college baseball team. Ryan is hindered by some tight hamstrings, which he continuously pulls because of how fast he can run. As the hamstrings tighten up more and more it starts to create dysfunction in the low back. When tested for range of motion, Ryan is one of the many unlucky chaps that can't even bend over and touch his toes. Ryan never worries about his movement. He lifts heavy weights and runs regularly, even though when he does so he is at the potential risk for injury. In Ryan's case we would say he has to work on his mobility (with a B) probably at the glute and hamstring location. Mobility is commonly defined as the ability to move freely or easily and even though it applies to the joints, is remedied mainly by just lengthening the muscles. I define mobility as, "Being able to exhibit strength through a functional range of movement while allowing an outlet for injury."

All of my programs are broken into two parts: goals, and missions. For the purpose of this book, we will have several mobility goals, but the mission is to be motile, or to be able to move spontaneously and actively.

3 Keys to Success

In order for motility to be restored to our low back, we must adhere to 3 major keys when performing our mobility exercises. These keys are placement, modality, and time.

Placement is often the most overlooked aspect of mobility work. Many people think that the area that is hurting (the low back in this instance) is where they need to place the foam roller, or the ball in order to get relief. This couldn't be further from the truth and in most cases is way off the mark. Sonja was having pain in her lower right side back and it was raveling down her right leg. I advised her to lie on her right side and put pressure on the Gluteus Minimus muscle to release it. She proceeded to lie on her back and roll around on the ball in the general area, but not where I specifically told her. She hopped up after two minutes and told me it still felt the same. I told her that's because she did not place the ball correctly. Trying again, I instructed her better and when she placed the ball correctly started to feel instant relief. Pain is often just the symptom and if you continuously treat the symptom, all you will do is continuously treat! You will never heal. I am trying to provide a permanent solution for you. Sometimes I will be telling you to press somewhere that may seem completely unrelated to your pain or symptoms, but it may be the dysfunction of this particular muscle that is causing the pain in your back. I will bring more clarity to this in the next chapter, but for now I invite you to be curious and perplexed when I tell you we will treat some areas of your body where the pain isn't and you will get a tremendous amount of relief from it!

Our second key to success is modality. I realize it is yet another similar sounding word, but this one has a tremendous amount of importance. Disrupting muscle tissue is no easy task. This is one of the many reasons those comfy white foam rollers and tennis balls don't really do the trick. It is theorized that our IT band, a muscle in the outer thigh running from the hip to the knee, could support the weight of a Volkswagen Beetle. Expecting a major change through the use of a tennis ball is like shooting a BB gun at a tank. I've had plenty of people tell me they have used softballs and tennis balls to loosen up their glutes to no avail. The reason why they do not get any relief is because the tennis ball is too soft, and the softball is too large. When I recommend a modality, it is okay to build up to it if the original modality is causing too much pain. Once the pain response lessens, we need to move on to the next step to allow for more specificity.

The more we can pinpoint or get on top of these trigger points and adhesions, the better. Everything will be spelled out for you in the chapters to come.

The third key to success is time. In 2013, an article in the Journal of The American Osteopath Association concluded that a minimum of 2 minutes of continuous foam rolling or consistently applied pressure needed to occur in order for the body to produce hyaluronic acid which is a natural oil that helps lubricate your muscles so they glide better and avoid getting stuck. Most people roll an area for 30 seconds and give up, moving on to their general workout. Some people may reach a solid minute if they are not paying attention, but the fact remains that time is another huge key to success. In some instances, I will only require you to roll an area for 3-5 minutes, and in others it may be a full 10-12! If 2 minutes is the bare minimum then we will only achieve the bare minimum results if that is how long we work. I want your results to be extraordinary, and after much experimentation have found my time recommendations to be both effective and efficient.

There you have it. When going through your restorative routine, remember to keep these three keys in mind for optimal results. Remember though, everything is scalable. If you can't take direct pressure on a muscle you can work around it, upstream or downstream. If a lacrosse ball isn't tolerable, move to a baseball, or a softball, and lastly if 3 minutes straight of pressure is too much try 30 second increments, resting for 10-20 seconds in between until your recommended time is reached.

The Kaizen Principle

The work you are about to embark on is difficult. This restorative motility program is for anyone, but not for everyone. If you were, or are an athlete you will be used to the discomfort these exercises cause. For those of you who believe all pain is bad pain you may find the program to be a bit of a challenge. Like I said earlier, we have to change the way our brain thinks about pain. Not all pain is destructive to the body. As long as you are not producing bruising, or levels of discomfort above 8 on your pain scale, it's more than likely the pain you are feeling is not only due to the unhealthy nature of the tissue but is also an indicator you are in the correct area for its release. It's at times like these that I ask you to be more aware of your body. I realize everyone is looking for the silver bullet or one stop shop but the time tested approach I am going to share with you is built off of what I call the *Kaizen* principle.

The Kaizen principle is a Japanese principle of business that states small improvements over time will make a large difference in the nature of your success. It is process focused, rather than results focused. Focusing on small improvements makes the program easier to implement. Depending on the nature of your pain and how it has developed in your body you may have to spend more time on some steps than you do on others. You may have to repeat some steps, or you may be able to skip one altogether. Some days we may feel significantly better than others. This doesn't mean we stop releasing and reeducating the area, it simply means we achieved a favorable response and continue as planned with the progression. In some instances, you may have a setback. This doesn't mean we are doing anything wrong, or that you injured yourself. Oftentimes the body has to heal in a reverse order, meaning it will get worse before it gets better. All of my clients have gotten significantly better after a setback and I now condition all of my current clients/athletes to expect them as a part of the healing process. I teach them to view it as a positive occurrence rather than a negative as the path to health is never a continuously ascending line. We will always move forward in increments.

How Long Will This Take?

The length of time it takes to heal oneself has many different factors to take into account. The first is how long has the pain been around? If you have been in pain for 1-3 months, I find usually 3-4 weeks of rolling will provide relief. That doesn't mean you don't have to stretch or do the exercises, but because the pain is fairly new and in the developmental stage still, it is easier to reverse. Typically if any adhesions or trigger points have developed they are easily disrupted and broken up with my methods. For those who have been in pain for over 3 months, but under 8 months I find 4-6 weeks of rolling and stretching consistently will provide tremendous relief. Stretching now becomes necessary because it is likely we have adhesions, which means our muscle tissue is stuck to itself.

The myofascial stretching we will do pulls the cross bridges apart and gets the muscle to open up and slide again restoring its length, decreasing the pain response. Lastly, for those who have been in pain for longer than 8 months especially surpassing a year, I typically shooting for a 2-3 month return to health time. You will have to roll and stretch extensively, and well as be very adamant with the complex of exercises I recommend to reeducate your glutes, hamstrings, and low back. When we operate in dysfunction for such long periods of time, we not only have to break the tissue up, and pull it apart, but we also need to teach the muscles how to fire correctly again when we move. The key to all of this is consistency—making sure you never take a day off! Your body will want to resist the changes you are making because you are disrupting the harmony it has created. It has created a balance in an imbalanced state and now you are trying to reverse that. Every movement you make, your body will want to tighten up what you loosened. By being consistent with this program, your muscles and nerves will restore their natural balance and thus reduce your pain. The next chapter will go into great detail about what that balance actually is.

Ask the Coach: What Makes This Different from Other Approaches?

This is a great question and one I truly enjoy answering. There are so many back pain remedies out there, it is extremely easy for the uneducated consumer to get confused. The reason why this approach is different is because I use many different techniques. An acupuncturist, for instance, will use needles to adjust energy meridians in the body. A massage therapist will only try to relax the muscles and not adjust the spine. A chiropractor will primarily adjust the spine, but not really release any tight muscles. What I do with my approach is cover three main areas of concern and that is releasing muscles that are producing pain in the low back or adjacent muscles, stretch those muscles to return them to their normal length so they stop affecting the bone in a negative manor, and then teach the muscles to fire correctly with strength training exercises so the pain does not come back and we truly correct the problem.

Chapter 4 - An Intricate Marriage

"Disease is the warning, and therefore the friend - not the enemy - of mankind."
–Dr. George S. Weger

Tom was a competitive bodybuilder for quite some time. He never really trained for the national competitions; rather he just stuck to the local ones, but was competitive nonetheless. With his days of competing behind him, he still hit the gym pretty hard as staying in shape was deeply ingrained in him by now. The day Tom got hurt was just like any other. He slept great, ate well, warmed up, and started to hit the weights when he noticed a disturbingly sharp pain in his left lower back. His body seized up and Tom was left there lying on the floor wondering what had happened. Tests and MRIs showed three disk herniations. Therapy wasn't helping. Tom couldn't sleep, sit, lie, or stand without incredible pain. He ended up finding me through a business associate of ours.

The day Tom came to see me, I could already see the problem the minute he got out of his car and started walking towards me. His right foot was facing straight ahead, and his left foot was turned out at 75 degrees. Tests showed extreme left glute tightness, and extreme right hip flexor tightness; he had what we call in physiology a lower-cross syndrome.

Utilizing our mobility and motility drills, we loosened up Tom's left glute with some rolling on a lacrosse ball followed by the proper stretches. Next, we had Tom roll on his right hip flexor to loosen it up, followed by the hip flexor stretch you are going to learn later in this book. Reversing a lower cross syndrome is all about time because it is a rotational problem. Because your body works in a spiral/rotational pattern, as you loosen the pattern up it will start to get tight again when you start to move. While this particular case was not a quick fix, Tom was pain free in three months' time and still enjoys pain free exercise to this day.

We Don't Know What We Don't Know

After my 30th birthday, I told myself I was going to stop lifting heavy, give my joints a break and start doing more marathons and triathlons. I did this for about three years and in that time went through about 6 bikes. The first one wasn't light enough, the second didn't have the right components, and the third had some aluminum instead of being all carbon. After every race I became more and more unsatisfied with my bike time so I kept switching out the bike. Finally, after taking my bike in for a tune-up one day, the mechanic asked me if I ever had my bike fitted to me and I said, "No, what is that?" He explained it is a service they offer where they adjust everything on my bike to optimize it for me to be as fast as possible. It was $80 and compared to the cost of a new bike at $3000 I guessed that it was a good idea. After having my bike fit for me, I had my best bike split ever in my next race.

What does this story illustrate? The entire time I was blaming my bike for being slow, it wasn't my bike, it was the fact I didn't know how to ride a bike. More specifically I didn't know how to optimize my bike for performance and this led to a lot of wasted time, and money on my part.

The first concern I always hear from my clients/athletes is, "I don't know why my back hurts." I tell them it's because they don't know how the back works. The purpose of this chapter is to help you understand what *you don't know you don't know* about how the back functions, and what an *intricate marriage* the muscles that comprise your midsection are in. Upset one of these bad boys and it's the back that suffers. Armed with this knowledge, we can better understand our condition, which will then help us to better treat ourselves.

Your Feet Tell All

In my opinion, Ida Rolf is the Godmother of pain management. In her amazing book *Rolfing: Reestablishing the natural alignment and structural integration of the human body for vitality and well-being,* she says, "Only by bringing peace from the ground up, can problems higher in the body be understood." So if we want to fully understand our back pain, we first need to look at our feet. If you ever go to the mall, or the beach, or any one large area where people congregate, I want you to look down and watch how people walk. Where are their feet facing? Where are your feet facing? More than likely they are facing out and this is where problem numero uno is.

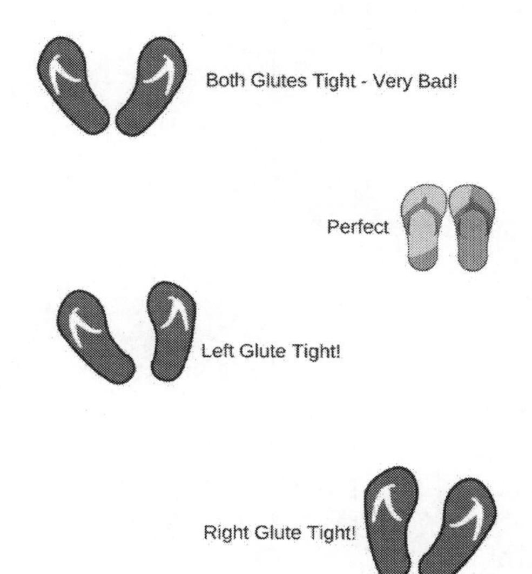

If you remember in chapter one I said we humans are machines, but we are not robots. If a robot is broken, that area just wore out too fast, that's all. With the human body being a web, if one area, in this case our feet, is not functioning correctly, this will largely affect the area that is translating the force the feet are producing. In this case, you guessed it: it's our back! Regardless if one foot or both feet are turned out, the back feels the dysfunction in the form of pain. The ankle and the knee are hinge joints meaning they function best through straightforward flexion and extension. By turning the foot out, the ankle becomes strained, the knee becomes strained, and the thigh now has to rotate in order to move forward.

Where could this car go?

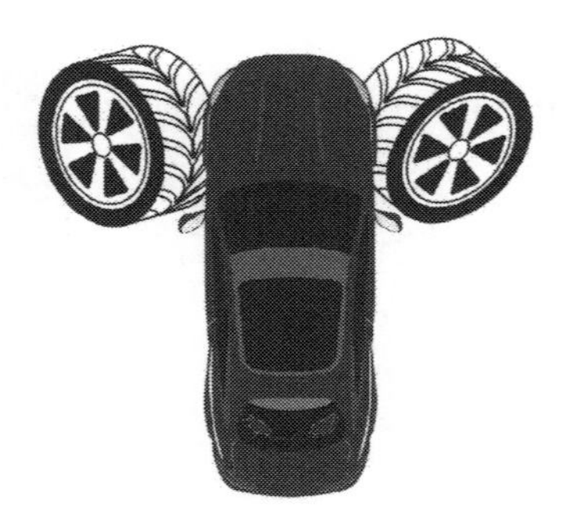

We need to understand that as human beings we walk with our low back, abdominals, and hip flexors, *on* our legs. We do not walk *with* our legs! When we are not pointing our feet in the direction of our movement, the back muscles will suffer. The back muscles simply were not designed for such wear and tear.

Being conscious of our foot position is the first step in eradicating our back pain. You can do everything else in this book to the best of your ability, but if you do not fix your foot position the pain will return. It's just that simple. An exercise I used to do in my gym was called walking Wednesday. I instructed all of my athletes to take their shoes off and walk feet forward for 3-5 minutes. Correcting your feet will take more than just 3-5 minutes, but it's a start. I recommend to walk barefoot as much as possible to allow you to actually feel what proper movement is like. It's also a great stimulus for your feet and helps ground us to the earth which syncs our sleep cycle. The second consideration we need to be aware of is our footwear. The lower the drop and the harder the sole the better. "But wait Chris, I need arch support!" No you don't, and you'll learn more towards the end of this book about why.

Your foot has not one, not two, but three arches, 26 bones, 33 joints, 109 ligaments, and 19 muscles and tendons. I'd say that's some decent support! Inhibiting the expansion and contraction of our foot's arch sends the wrong signal to the rest of our body from the ground up. In my experience, the best types of shoes have a very hard sole, and have a 3-4 degree drop. If you like zero drop shoes then go for it. Shoes that have high heels combined with cushiony air, or gel may be comfortable for your feet, but strain these mechanisms we depend on to move. Depending on which type of shoes you decide to buy, we need to be aware that a lower drop in the sole of the shoe will increase foot activity, which will increase calf activity as well. If you're a runner, be careful to not start off too quickly or you'll wake up the next day with some pretty tender calf muscles!

A question I pose to my clients is, "Can you start today?" If you can't go buy new shoes today, can you start walking with your feet forward today? Surely there's nothing stopping you from doing that. Like I said earlier, there is no magic bullet, no miraculous cure. Just a bunch of little changes we are going to make that will produce big results!

Your Sacred Seat: The Hip Flexors

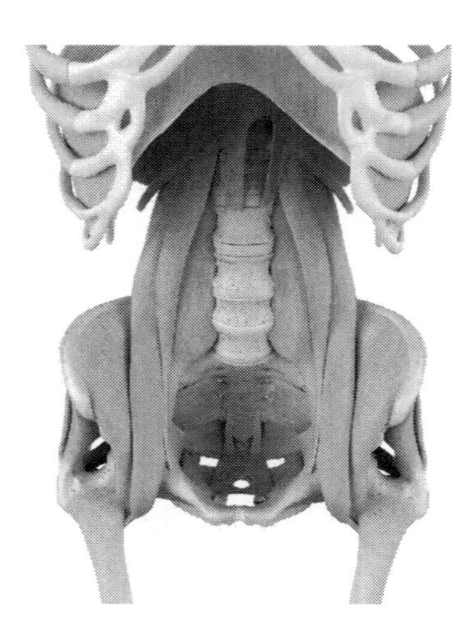

Your pelvis is actually referred to in anatomy as your sacred seat. The sacred seat I am referring to is the one you are sitting on right now! Sitting is quickly becoming the new smoking and has been found to have many links to heart disease, and even cancer. In Jo Ann Staugaard-Jones' book The Vital Psoas Muscle: *Connecting physical, emotional, and spiritual well-bei*ng she wrote about a case study where 12 adult volunteers recorded sitting for a minimum of 5 hours on good days to a maximum of 11 hours on bad days! Sitting is a destroyer of the proper function of your psoa and illiacus muscles, which are more commonly called your hip flexors. Your hip flexors are at their longest which is about 16 inches in length when you are standing up. When seated they shorten considerably. Remaining in this position causes your hip flexors to lock in a shorter position than they can function well in. This causes not only back pain (they originate at the 12th thoracic vertebrae which is the major rotational joint in the back to the 5th lumbar vertebrae, descending down and attaching to your femur) but can also create problems with our breathing and circulation as well.

Continuing with our fascial web ideology, what we find with the hip flexors is even more amazing. The fascia from our hip flexors continues along and connects to our diaphragm, our heart, our lungs, our kidneys, and several other organs. Having dysfunctional or tight hip flexors not only means our back will hurt from its improper length, but our respiration will suffer, as well as our hearts ability to pump blood. Those are two key elements I just don't want to change in my body, if you ask me! Since locomotion is first initiated with your hip flexors, it makes no wonder that they are also directly linked to your brain's fight or flight response. Chronic negative thinking puts your hip flexors in a chronically contracted state. This negative feedback loop can in some cases create severe anxiety, and is also why many believe that your emotions have a huge correlation with back pain. The healing methods we will be using for the hip flexors are not very comfortable and I urge you to take them on slowly, but neglecting these muscles will also, once again, not allow you to heal your back pain fully. There are going to be days where you will want to take the day off from those exercises, but those will be the days that will benefit you the most!

I know what you are thinking: "What can I do to start right now?!?!" I have my athletes and clients abide by the 20/20 rule. Every 20 minutes you are sitting, stand up and do something for 20 seconds. Do a squat, walk to the water fountain, go to the fridge, or even stand up and do some light stretching – just don't get stuck in that position!

Your Abs Are Not Your Core

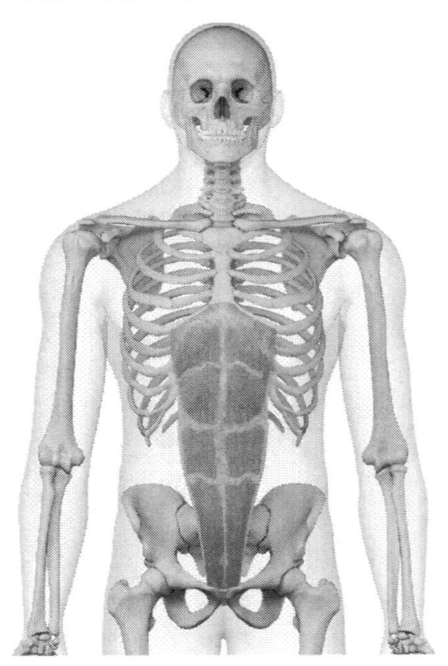

Who doesn't love the way a chiseled six-pack looks on a handsome man or woman? It's been labeled as the holy grail of fitness in some circles. You can have chicken legs and a spaghetti back, weigh 110 pounds soaking wet, but if you have a six-pack you must be fit! I hate to break it to you guys, but in 18 years of coaching I have never done a single abdominal exercise that helped me run faster, lift heavier, or jump higher, and when my back was hurting doing anything abs related was the furthest from my mind. Yet we live in a culture that glorifies the abdominals and we have practitioners who tell people their back pain is stemming from ab weakness and advise them to do "core exercises," which translates to a bunch of sit ups. Sit-up type of exercises can be disastrous for those who have tight hip flexors because the hip flexors will initiate most of the movement. You are now working chronically tight and stressed out hip flexors even harder thus persisting your back pain. A simple stretching of the hip flexors, combined with a strengthening of the lower lumbar muscles, glutes, and hamstrings is a much more effective option. Now does this mean we totally neglect the abdominal muscles and never train them? No! Every muscle in the body should be trained to be strong and effective, sit-ups and direct abdominal training is simply not the best way to get rid of your back pain.

Your real "core" is what I call your hip flexors, quadratus lumborum (lower back muscle), gluteal (butt) muscles, and your hamstrings (back of the thigh muscle). Take one of those muscles away and you take away your movement. Think about it – nobody calls into work sick with sore abdominals. No one says, "This chair is really killing my abs." Tight hip flexors bring your head closer to your hips, rendering the abdominals ineffective at supporting your organs, and your lower back. Strengthening them without addressing your tight hip flexors will not improve your posture or position. Oh, and one last thing, *stop referring to them as your core*!

You Don't Have Back Pain, You Have a Butt Problem

You have heard me refer to these mysterious muscles known as the "glutes" for a while now. If you knew what I was talking about – great, this will expand your knowledge. If you had no idea what I was talking about, you are in for a treat! The glutes are comprised of three muscles: the gluteus minimus, gluteus medius, and gluteus maximus. To make things more interesting we have four parts to our gluteus maximus, which are the lateral part of the lateral, the medial part of the lateral, the lateral part of the medial, and the medial part of the medial. We will learn how to target these areas in our strengthening section. The primary point we need to understand in this section is how our glutes affect the function of our low back. When we take a step, muscular force is not transferred straight up the body, rather when it reaches the glute of the side that the foot is in contact with the floor, it then crosses over to the other side of the back on up to the shoulder. To put it plainly, our bodies function in an X pattern, as illustrated in the diagram below:

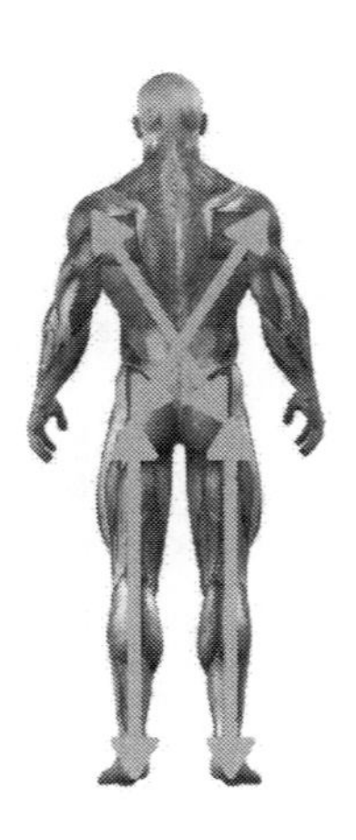

You can test this very easily if you want by walking with the backs of your hands on your lower back. Feel which side of your back contracts when you walk compared to which foot you have on the ground. When your left foot strikes the ground, you will feel a contraction in you right lower back, and when you right foot hits the ground you will feel a contraction in your left lower back. Having your body function this way is very efficient and allows for a smooth gait pattern. If the right glute and right low back fired at the same time we would all be walking like penguins and penguins do not walk very fast or very efficiently!

As we discussed earlier though, human beings do not move correctly 100% of the time. We all have faults, myself included and when we rely too much on one leg, or have trauma incurred on one side of the body, we develop a deficiency that will then hinder how our back functions. When the dysfunction first occurs, the back says, "Hey, no problem, I got this!" But after a couple of months or a couple of years depending on how much stress you put on your back, it will eventually come to a breaking point where pain is produced. Remember, your entire body's system is a yes man; it will keep doing what you ask of it till the structure no longer holds. When we start feeling pain, we have had a problem for some time, and this then takes time for us to reverse.

In most cases what happens is one glute will get tight, the other glute will get weak and the more unilaterally we become imbalanced the more taxing it becomes on the lower back. Close to 95% of all back pain cases I treat are cured by not even touching the back. We spend most of our time correcting our hips. When the hips are corrected, the stress on the back alleviates and you become a happy camper. Correcting the glutes is tricky as there are three separate areas we need to work on with absolute precision. Just rolling around on your butt without an objective will get you nowhere. With that said, let's take a close look at each one of these muscles starting with my favorite – the gluteus minimus.

The Gluteus Minimus

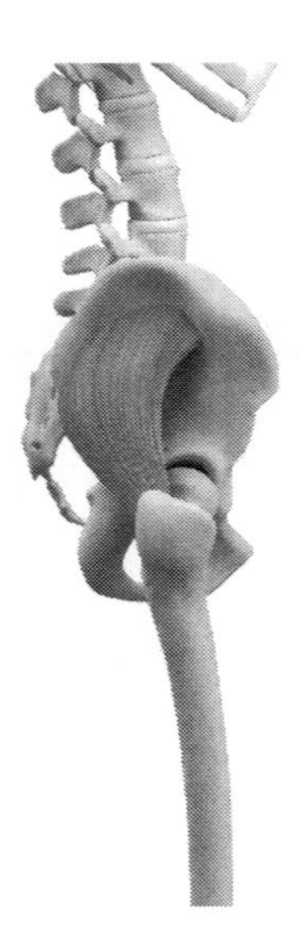

To get a feeling of what it is like when this muscles is tight, think about putting on a pair of pants that are two sizes too small for you. Then put a belt on and tighten that sucker as much as you can, sucking in your stomach even. Once all of that is accomplished, try bending over or even doing a simple squat. Impossible, right? That is the damage this little guy can cause. Many people will also suffer from what I call "Fake Sciatica" in which the subject will have pain radiating down their leg sometimes to their foot, yet their flexibility checks out. No tight hamstrings, no tight glute muscles, or hip muscles. These people are prescribed painkillers and muscle relaxers and sent on their way, when a little pressure at their hip would cure all. Too simple I suppose.

The gluteus minimus internally rotates your thigh, and also abducts it, which means it moves your leg away from the midline of your body. It is a very, very active muscle stabilizing the pelvis to the femur (thigh bone) and contracts every time you shift your weight from side to side. Shifting your weight to one leg while standing will stress this guy out, so will long trips in planes, trains, and automobiles. Releasing it can be very entertaining because of where it will send pain. It is somewhat of a rogue muscle in that respect, but when we do get it to release it will feel like you squirted a quart of oil in your back!

The Gluteus Medius

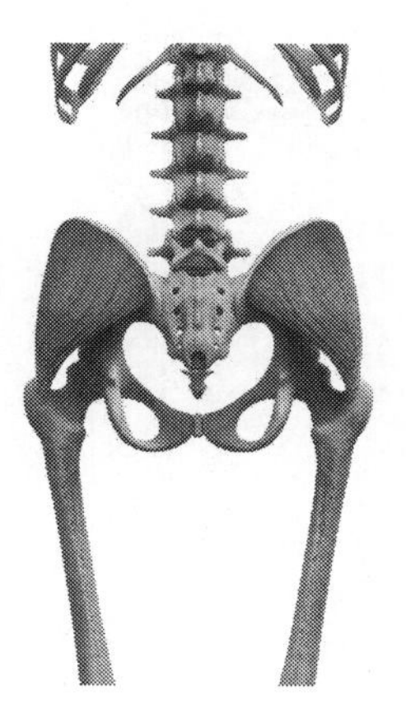

The gluteus medius muscle—as you can see by where it originates and where it inserts—can hugely affect the health of our back. If one side decides to get tighter than the other, our pelvis will become uneven and BOOM! We have back pain. The gluteus medius wears many hats. It helps to flex and internally rotate the hip, as well as extends and externally rotates the hip. It also abducts the leg (moving it away from the midline of the body) as well as stabilizes the pelvis when shifting weight (i.e. placing all of your weight on one leg while waiting in line at Macy's). We can develop trigger points in the gluteus medius that will send pain right into our lower back and coccyx region. This guy will also refer a lot of pain down into the hamstring as well and can be very tender to even lay a finger on, but doing so will reap big rewards lessening our back and hip pain.

The Gluteus Maximus

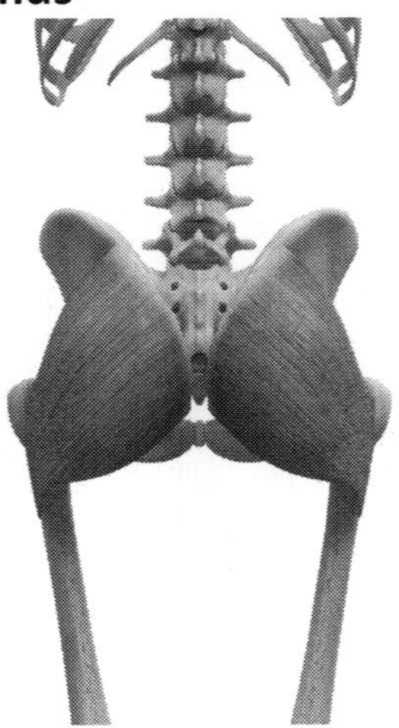

Development of the gluteus maximus is what has allowed human beings to stand upright and separate us from our primate ancestors. The gluteus maximus is one of the strongest muscles in the body and also consumes the most calories when being activated but you wouldn't know it looking at contemporary American society. As an outsider looking in you would think it was just a large pad to cushion our pelvis as we sit all day long in various seats of either modalities of transportation or workspaces. While it does not contain any trigger points that will actively cause back pain, neglecting to stimulate the gluteus maximus muscle will cause it to atrophy (decrease in size), and weaken which will place more stress on the lower back muscles to keep the spine erect. Case in point, you never see an elderly person who has C-spine and large gluteus muscles. Their back literally blends in with their tush!

The primary gig of the gluteus maximus is to extend the hips, which makes it a prime mover in walking and standing from a seated position. I hope you like your rump nice and hot because we will be doing plenty of exercises that will stimulate it in ways you never thought possible!

The Hamstrings

The Hamstring Group

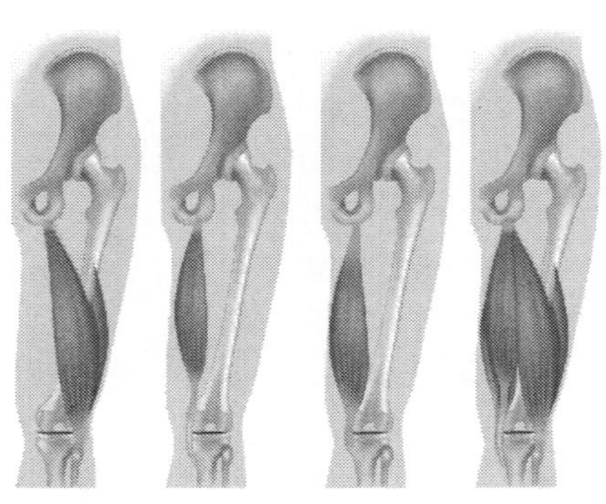

Technically called the biceps femoris, the hamstrings, have not two, not even three, but four muscles as you can see in the picture. I think it was one of those times where we may have named something before we actually studied it, but I digress. The hamstrings are important because they are called upon second to help the glutes do their job before the back is. The correct firing order is glute first, ipsilateral (same side) hamstring second, contralateral (opposite side) low back muscles third. When the hamstring is tight, or weak and not doing its job properly, who do you think picks up the slack? Your good old friend the low back, that's who. Frequent and prolonged sitting can easily create trigger points in your hamstrings, tightening them more and more, rendering them completely useless. Doing a yoga class or two may show signs of improvement, but continued stretching of trigger point laden hamstrings will only tighten and compress the knots which will then start sending pain into the calf muscle leaving practitioners really confused and you really frustrated. We need pressure to release the trigger points; only then can we start to stretch them and return them to a happy length.

Bonus: The Deep Muscles of the Pelvis

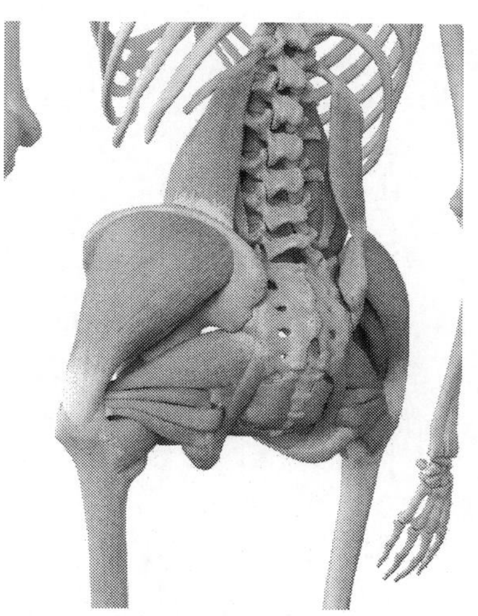

While not contributors to too much back pain, the deep muscles are worth noting because if they are tight, they will cause the foot to turn out in our no-no duck walking fashion. Traditional tests for glute tightness will check out okay, but subjects will only be able to achieve partial ranges of motion in a squat at best. Forcing beyond a 90-degree knee position in a squat will be impossible unless one turns their feet out sharply. This will cause a tremendous amount of instability at the knee, and way more than normal hip flexion in order to get down deep enough. Access to these guys is tough because of the thickness of the gluteus maximus and is best addressed by a manual therapist. This doesn't mean you can't roll a lacrosse ball on them in your spare time though and get acquainted. I call them generically your deep rotators, but here are their specific names:

Piriformis – most of you have heard of this guy because when he tightens, he puts pressure on the sciatic nerve, which is not so fun.
Superior and Inferior Gemellus – These guys laterally rotate your thigh. When these tighten, your foot position will become altered to the dreaded duck position.
Obturator Internus – Laterally rotates femur (pointing the toes out again!)
Quadratus Femoris – Another lateral rotator of the thigh and hip stabilizer.

Although this section may seem pretty straightforward, there are plenty of gems hidden in here. The better you understand this chapter, the better you will be able to sense your own tightness and ultimately your own path to wellness. Without further adieu, let's get to the fun stuff now!

Ask the Coach: What About Icing My Back?

Without any of this prior knowledge I made one of the greatest mistakes of my life when my back was hurt. I actually used heat, not ice. With all the confusion surrounding my injury I reduced myself to electrical stim treatments in the athletic training room, and combined it with some stretches I found on the Internet. I would do these twice a day, after my 6 a.m. women's basketball team, and then before I exercised (upper body only obviously) at 4 p.m. The reason I used heat was simple;

for comfort. Who wants a massive bag of ice thrown on their back at 7 in the morning? After the first day I used ice I got up from the table and started walking stiff as a board – my back almost hurt more! When I switched to heat however, it was not only more comfortable, but when I stood up from the table I couldn't believe how loose my back felt. As a budding young physiologist, rather than overthinking the situation, I just went with what felt better. Surely I'm not just telling you to stop using ice based off of a feeling? Nope, I'm sure not!

In November of 2005 an athlete of mine had a received word that the Chicago Bears were coming down to watch him practice and then play in the upcoming season finale game against nationally ranked Washington State. The problem was the scouts from the Bears were coming down to see him Thursday, and he had just twisted his ankle badly in practice on Monday. He called me in a panic and I quickly took to the World Wide Web to find a quick, reliable solution.

All of my research led me to a book by Coach Dick Hartzell, the creator of Jump Stretch Bands who wrote a book called *Don't Ice That Ankle Sprain!* In the book, Coach Hartzell explains how ice constricts blood vessels, restricting blood flow to the ankle as it tries to heal. He recommended heat, and some mobility work with bands in order to free up the ankle from its injury and help return its much-needed proprioception. The technique worked like a charm. My athlete hobbled into my apartment, and after about an hour of the band work and some light massage around the calf and ankle, he was sprinting at 90% capacity up and down my hallway. I was amazed.

If you haven't gotten the feeling by now, let me come right out and tell you – I'm a physiology rebel! I don't really like tradition, or following in someone else's footsteps. I want to be on the cutting edge of treatment, or blazing a path for others to follow. I love debunking myths and succeeding where others with more illustrious credentials have failed. I've had my athletes and patients practice what I have taught them in a public gym and they always come back to me and tell me how someone with some kind of certification told them what they are doing to their shoulder/knee/back etc. is not good for them. I instruct those who work with me to politely say, "Thank you for the help," and never to argue with them. They don't know what they don't know, and it's not their fault.

I now never use ice in any situation except post injury, or post operation to 12 hours after and in the knee only. All other situations I instruct people to use heat and mobility, or self-applied massage only and here's why: In 2012, a study in the British Journal of Sports Medicine showed that there is no clinical evidence ice improves the healing of muscle strains. Consequently, there was also a study published in the 2013 Journal of Strength and Condition Research showing that icing can actually hinder recovery from eccentric muscle work. In another 2013 study involving eleven 20-year-old male baseball players, topical cooling caused a significant increase in muscle damage markers during recovery from eccentric exercise. All of the pictures you see of athletes jumping in ice baths post workout, or post game seem silly now doesn't it? In all honesty it should be illegal. A 20-million-dollar-a-year athlete doing damage to his body willingly! Let us continue though.

A research study published in 2012 by the Journal of Sports Medicine showed that in 25 separate studies, 75% of them reported a decrease in muscular strength following icing. There was also evidence from six studies that cooling adversely affected speed, power, and agility-based running tasks. So when Jimmy, the high school running back, bangs his knee, gets a pile of ice thrown on it, and then returns to the game like a champ, we are asking for further injury to the area.

Icing is really just a great placebo effect. It is great at decreasing pain—no doubt—but in the process we are not letting our body heal correctly. When an injury occurs, the body's repair mechanism comes in the form of inflammation, which contains all of the healing components. Why do we want to decrease the availability of these healing components by using ice and shunning inflammation? Why do we think our wisdom is greater than 4 million years of evolution? As I said before, the only time ice should be permitted is post-operation when inflammation needs to be controlled due to the invasive process of surgery. All other injuries should be heated to increase circulation and nerve conductivity (researchers believe ice slows down nerve impulses), mobilized in a somewhat pain-free manner, and continuously massaged to prevent the formation of scar tissue and help move along the process of draining the inflammation into the lymph nodes.

We also find out in an article on caringmedical.com that peripheral blood perfusion can be reduced while icing which means that blood vessels constrict and shut off blood flow that brings in healing cells. Depending on the duration of the icing, it can take up to several hours for the blood vessels to open back up again. This can in effect cause the damaged tissue to die, and permanently damage the nerve. I don't know about you guys, but I like my nerves alive, not dead.

There is a gigantic difference between speculation and experimentation. I have had nothing but phenomenal results treating injuries, sore muscles, and joints, as well as post-op patients with heat, movement, and foam rolling for over 11 years now! So there you have it, you are under strict orders to get in the hot tub, or your favorite Swedish or infrared sauna to help relax your pain away. Leave the ice baths for the polar bears!

Chapter 5 – Step 1: Mobility

"All that man needs for health and healing has been provided by God in nature, the challenge of science is to find it." Philippus Theophrastrus Bombast that of Aureolus Paracelsus (1493-1541)

Annie came to me in pretty bad shape. Her pain was the result of poorly applied therapy after a bad car accident when she was on college. She was now 45 years old and her husband had to help her to walk from the car to come see me. Listening to Anne talk you could sense the fatigue and desperation in her tone. She was tired of her back going out on her leaving her in bed or on the couch for sometimes up to two weeks. She was tired of missing out on the days her husband would take their two kids to the beach or on the boat to wakeboard. She was tired of all the worry she had surrounding her movement everyday. She had lost her motility and the plethora of practitioners she has visited over the years made for a pretty impressive conversation over cocktails, but that was about it. Nobody could figure out how to help her. Was she broken? That's the first question she asked me. I assured her that as long as she could get to me she was not the least bit broken. "We are all different, but the same," I told her. We each have the same capacity for injury as we do to heal; we just need to be in the right care.

Careful inspection of Annie showed tightness in her right glute/hamstring complex, which carried up to her left shoulder. She had been favoring her left leg for 25 years! Through vigilant application of our mobility and motility exercises, Annie was pain free after four months and even became a member of my gym, dropping nearly 30 pounds and increasing her fitness to pre-college levels! Her story is one of my favorites to tell not because of the success we achieved, but because of the hardships she endured along the way.

People feel a return to health should always be an ascending line, and this may be the case if your pain is just developing.

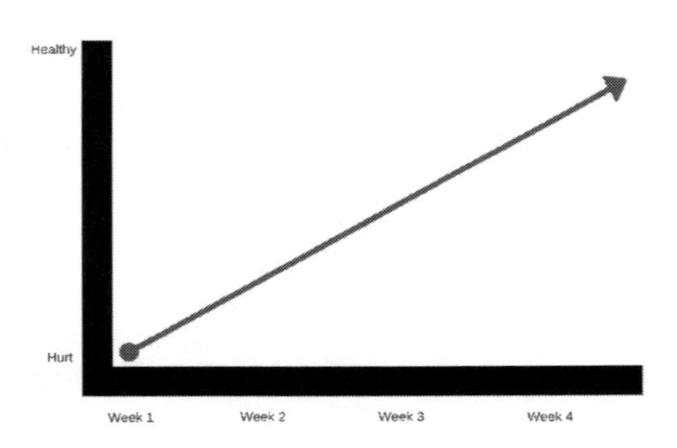

Sample timeline of a person with pain for less than 3 months.

When you have been in pain for as long as Annie had been, your return to health will look a little more like this:

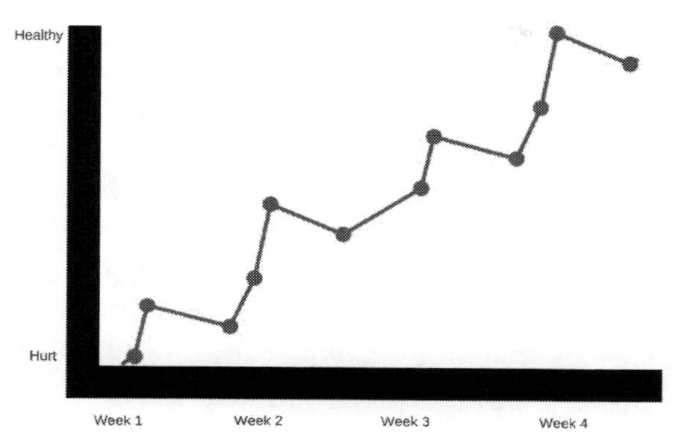

Did Annie have some setbacks? Absolutely! And I told her to expect them. Her body had created what I call "functioning chaos," which meant anyway it could develop force for her to traverse the physical plane it did so at the expense of her muscles, tendons, ligaments, and ultimately her joints. We had to break this chaos down and restore order to her movement. This neuromuscular reeducation will sometimes cause a spasm, or the brain to go on high alert. This is because we are making swift changes to the body's structure and if it does not calibrate just as quick, it will force you to slow your movement down. This is where our patience and persistence comes in. Even though we may be hurting, we are not hurting the body. I was providing a paradigm shift for Annie no other practitioner was willing to take her through. We adapted to her body's responses and adjusted our exercises accordingly to the imposed demands. As we slowly put her blocks back together, her brain, and central nervous system calmed down and stopped referring pain.

Called to Care

I love you. I love everyone who comes looking to me for care. That's why this book is dedicated to you, the reader. I know it sounds cliché or corny, but there were plenty of times in my life I was in pain and there was no one there to help me. Those who tried, tried diligently, but just didn't have the right answers and that's okay. Fixing me wasn't their calling, it was mine. I'm one of the lucky few who don't question why I'm here, or what my purpose is. I am constantly *called to care* for those who are looking to take their pain away for good. My success rate is dictated by holding the space for you to heal. With malpractice suits flying around like Boeing 747s these days, it's no wonder doctors and physical therapists shake their heads and send the tough cases packing. If someone is treating you based off of fear first, your treatment will be limited. I'm not saying all practitioners are like this, but it's safe to say some (if not a majority) are.

If you get anything out of this book know that I believe in you. I believe you are in pain, and I believe you want to be happy and healthy again, regaining your freedom of movement. While I do get stumped sometimes, our body will always show us signs of ways to heal it. Pay great attention because this could be as slight as a buzzing sensation, or in some cases may come as a loud crack or pop. Whatever the case is remember you always have me in your corner! Experience has shown me that some of the movements I teach in this book can be quite tricky to understand through just pictures and text. As a result I created a video library of all of the movements so you can follow along and better understand how to perform them. Included with the videos is also a three month program to help accelerate your success. If you feel this is something you may want to take advantage of, please email me at chris@influentialhealthsolutions.com and I will give you directions on how to do so!

In other cases there are some people that don't feel comfortable doing any of these exercises by themselves. I completely understand because the methods I put forth in this book are a completely new way of ridding pain not only in the lower back, but the entire body as well. That being said, if you would like a free consultation or to work one-on-one with me please e-mail me directly at chris@influentialhealthsolutions.com.

Abdominal Mobility

Remember how I told you that the abdominals are pretty much worthless when trying to heal your back? Well that wasn't entirely true. It is well documented that there are some pretty serious trigger points in your abdominals that refer pain directly into your back as indicated by the pictures below:

Trigger Point Locations

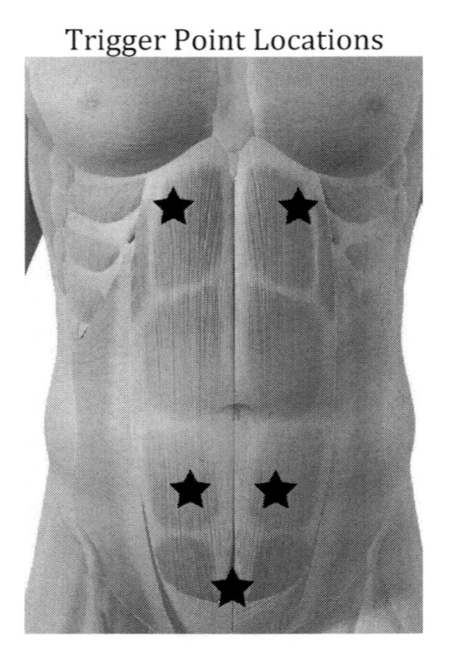

Back Pain Referral Pattern

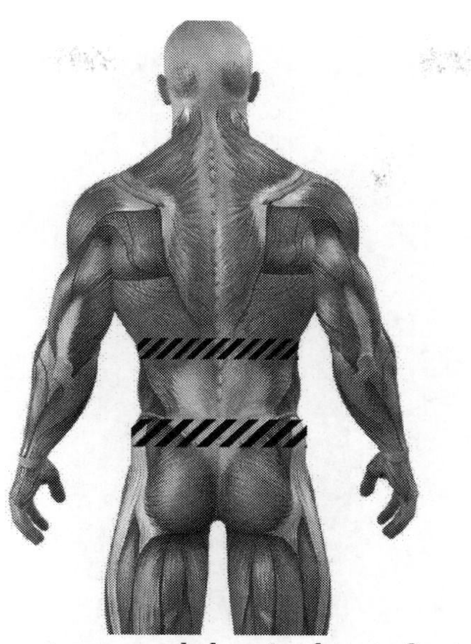

Rolling out your abdominals at first may seems strange and feel highly unpleasant, but I have had the most immediate relief in back pain, and increase in hamstring flexibility come as a result of doing so. This mobilization will pay off in big dividends and that is why I am putting it first. Here is your model for releasing your abdominal trigger points:

Method – Lying on your stomach placing direct pressure, or stirring the pot by rolling around searching for any tissue that sends pain into our back. Support yourself with your elbows or your hands, you do not want to swan dive on to the ball!

Modality – Softball.

Time – 6-10 minutes on the entire abdominal sheet!

Ball Placement

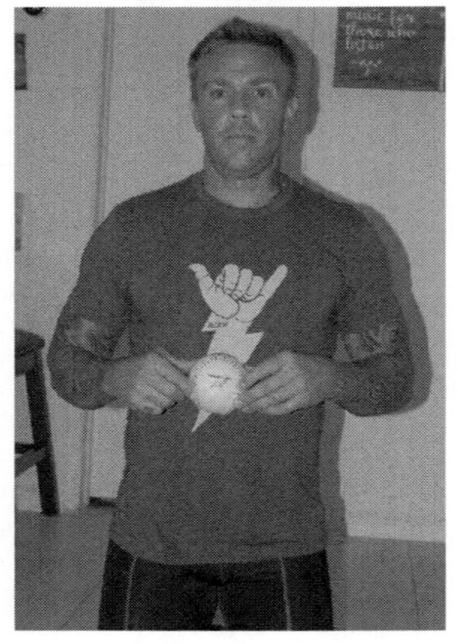

Lying on your stomach with elbow support

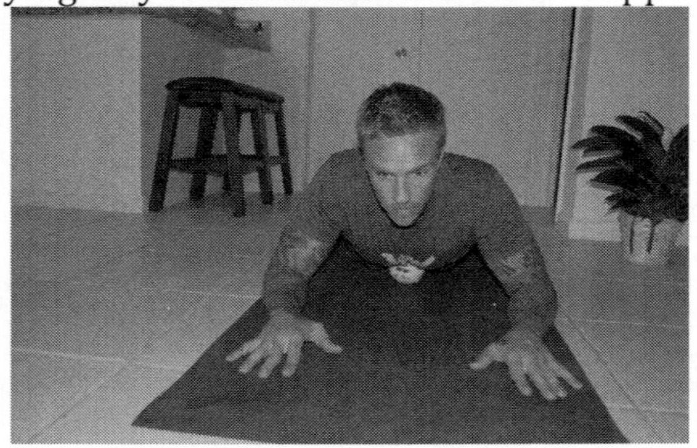

If your results are limited on the ground, you may want to try using the back of a chair, or sofa and leaning into the ball to apply deeper pressure:

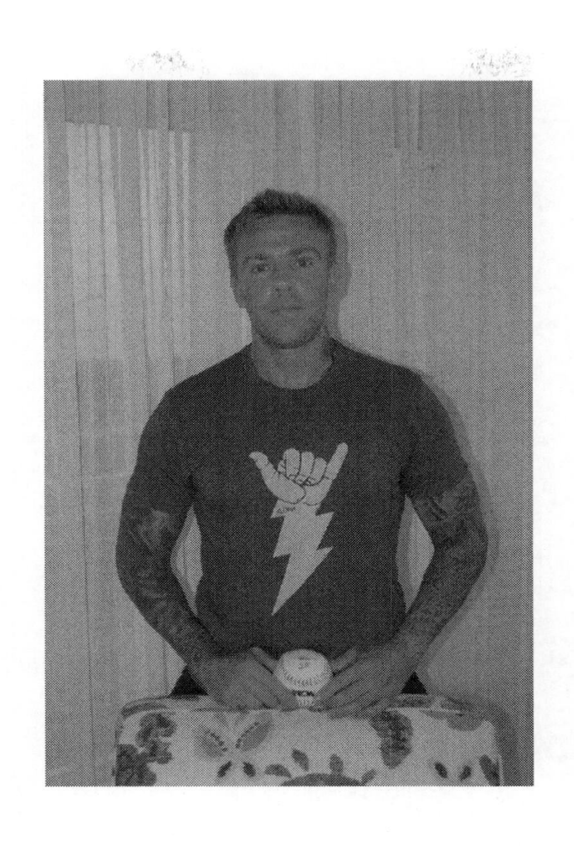

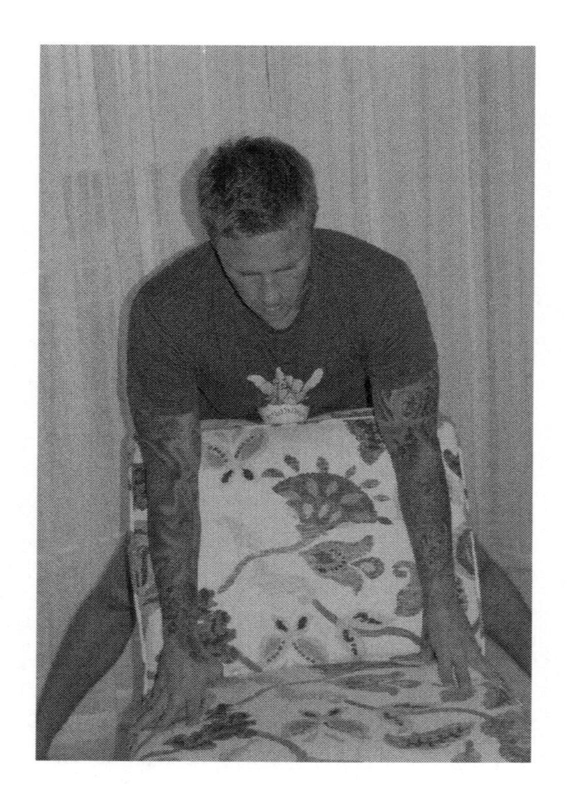

Trigger points are interesting due to the fact that they refer pain into seemingly unattached muscle groups. By now you, the reader knows this makes perfect sense because the body is a web and completely connected! By attacking the abdominal trigger points first, we loosen what may be causing the back to feel painful and tight before we roll the back, getting much more out of our back mobility exercises!

Hip Flexor Mobility

Such a critical muscle for not only support, but also vitality, you know we were going to go hunting around in here to lengthen and restore their proper function. The flexor trigger points are deep and very difficult to get to. Due to their depth they must be stimulated slowly and carefully. Here is your model:

Method – Lying flat on your stomach, place the ball at the lowest trigger point area. Once you have found the spot lift the same leg of the side the ball is on, and the opposite arm, supporting yourself with the opposite arm and leg still on the floor. Return your arm and leg to the floor and repeat as many repetitions as possible.

Modality – Softball.

Time: 2 minutes for each trigger point.

Trigger point location

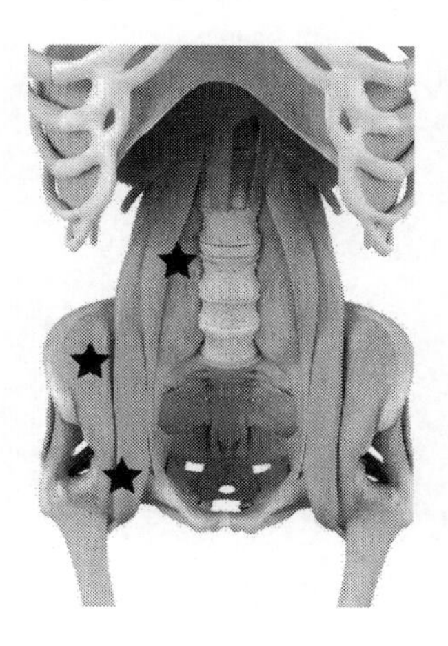

Back Pain Referral Pattern

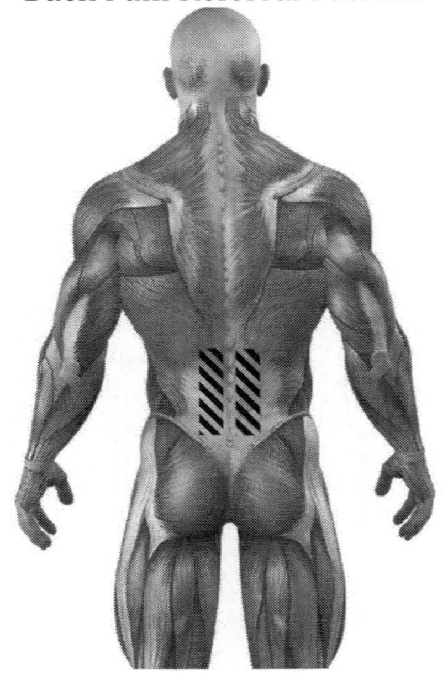

Ball Placement

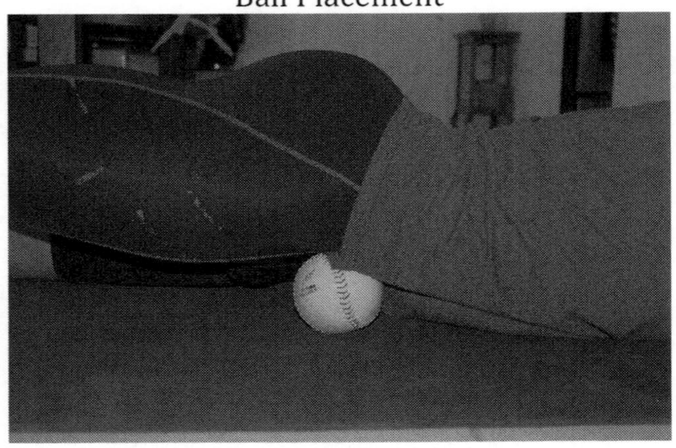

The ball is on my right hip flexor, so I raise my left arm

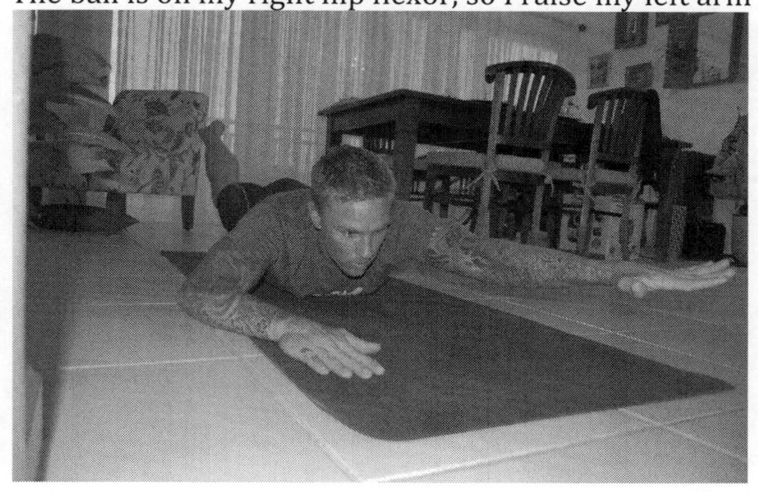

And my right leg

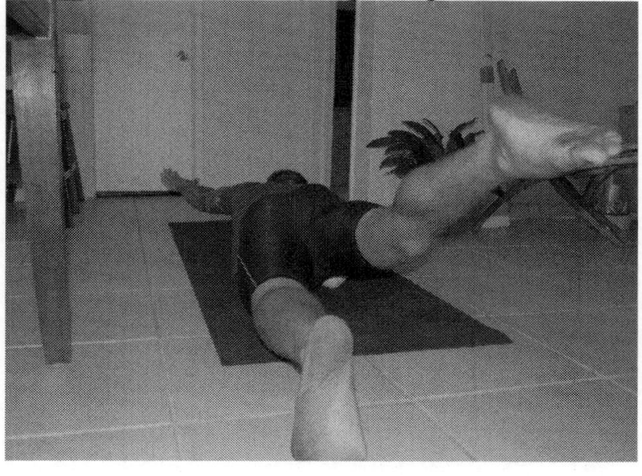

Be patient as we are using a pumping action to get the trigger points to release. If you feel comfortable enough while doing this mobilization, you can also relax and apply some direct pressure to it. This is common sense but needs to be stated. Your gut along with a lot of major organs lie close to your hip flexors, which should dictate caution on your part. Do not press into any area that is referring intense pain into your gut. If you are on the trigger point and it is a normal muscle soreness that is fine. If the pain is going into your back even better! These are both great mobilizations, but because of their sensitive nature not a lot of practitioners will advocate their use. I on the other hand have found way too many problems in these muscles to omit them, and still be able to sleep as soundly as I do. Bottom line is to be gentle, and use caution and you will produce a win-win for your back!

Gluteus Minimus Mobility

While most of the pain from a tight gluteus minimus will refer pain down the leg creating what I call "fake sciatica," it will feel as though there is an inability to bend over fully and a slight pull on the lower back. We kill two birds with one stone utilizing this mobilization. If the trigger points are active, you may feel pain traveling down your leg. If the muscle is only tight, then the mobilization will still be sore, and your back will feel a lot looser when you stand up. Here is your model:

Method - Lying completely on your side, place the ball at your belt line slightly under the top of your hipbone. Keep that same leg straight, and bend the opposite leg placing that foot on the floor. Allow all of your weight to sink into the ball on the gluteus minimus and focus on breathing to release and relax that muscle.

Modality – Ideally a lacrosse ball, but a baseball can be used at the beginning if a lacrosse ball is too sore.

Time – 4 minutes per side.

Gluteus Minimus Trigger Points

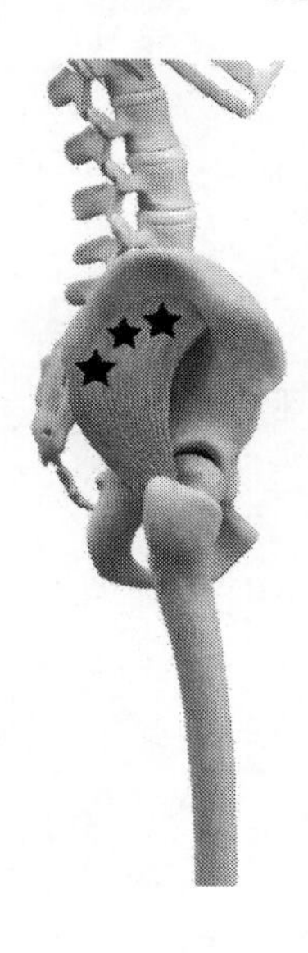

Ball placement

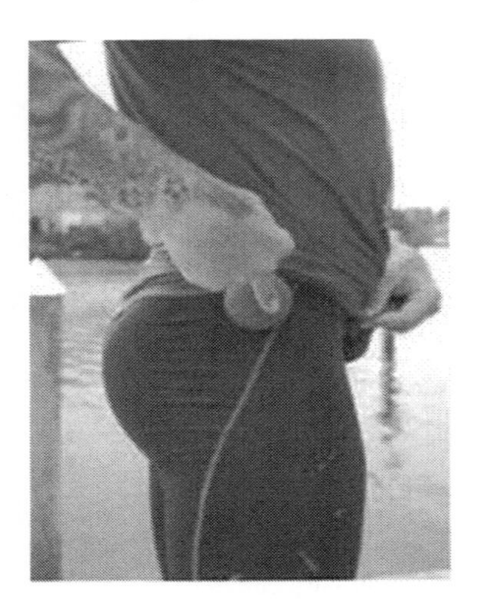

Lie on your side, opposite knee bent, and foot on the floor

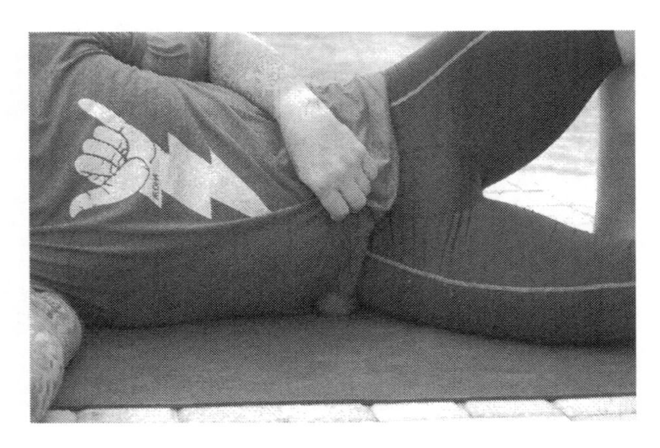

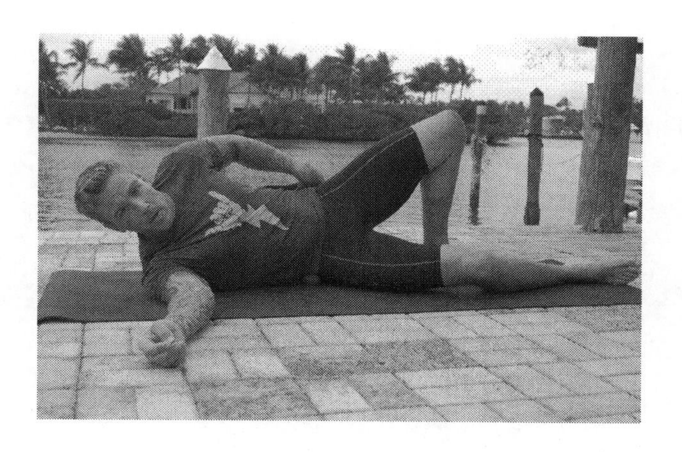

I can't over-emphasize how important this mobilization is, or how sore this overworked, and underappreciated muscle can be sometimes. Many people have never even heard of this muscle before, but never forget it again after their first time applying pressure to it. If the pain exceeds our 6-8 ranges, use a larger ball, or take breaks until you have achieved the prescribed amount of time.

Gluteus Medius Mobility

Flying low under the radar, gluteus medius trigger points can create a lot of pain in the back and the hamstring. This will cause both to feel tight and not function too well, which will prompt you to feel like you have to stretch them. Stretching will tighten the trigger points, but lengthen the muscle giving you a false positive which means you'll feel looser, but more pain will develop. Not good. Here's your model:

Method – Using a lacrosse ball, lie on your side like you are going to mobilize your gluteus minimus. From there, turn your body slightly and roll it along the crest of your hip where the trigger points are located in the diagram below. This is a somewhat funny position because you are not on your back and you are not directly on your side. You are in between both of those positions.

Modality – Ideally a lacrosse ball, but a baseball may be used at the beginning if the area is sore and referring pain above our 6-8 tolerance scale.

Time – 4-6 minutes for this bad boy!

Gluteus Medius Trigger Points

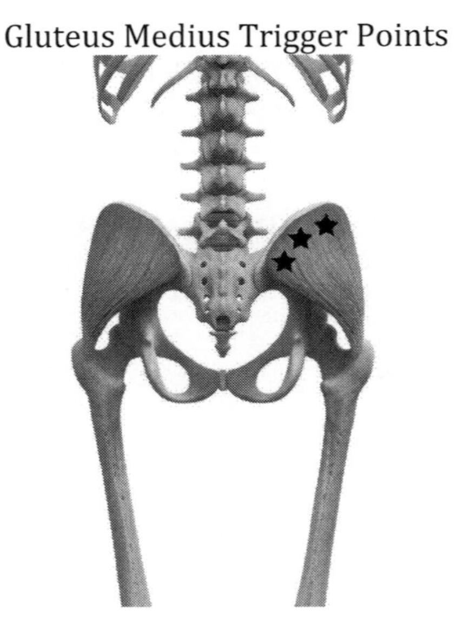

Back Pain Referral Pattern

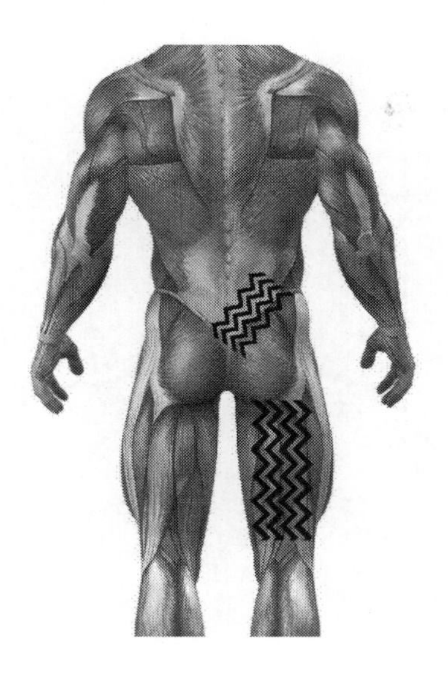

Ball position

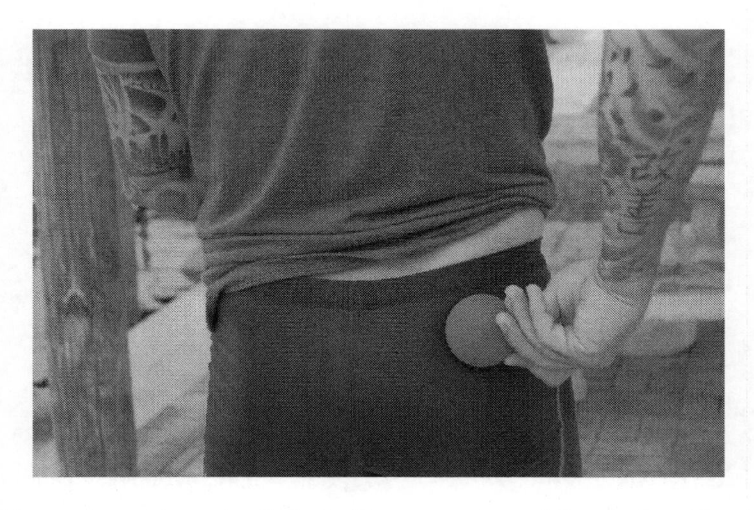

Lie on your side and roll the ball into position while not directly on your side and not directly on your back.

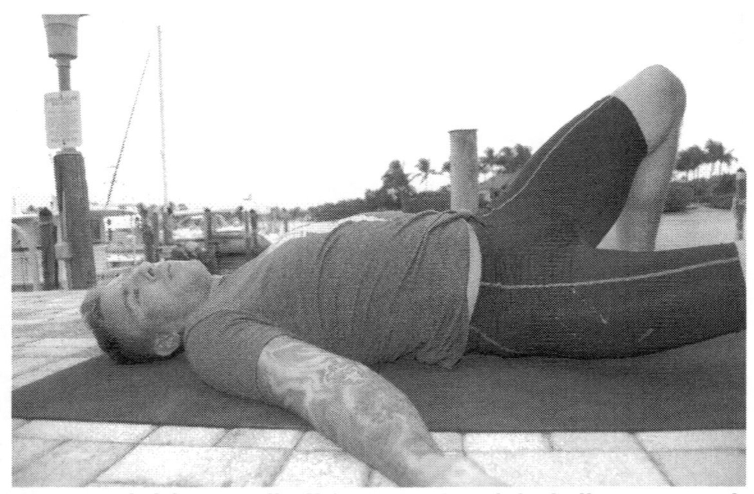

Notice, my left hip is still off the ground, and the ball is on my right gluteus medius.

A tender gluteus medius will present itself very quickly. You may experience some pain traveling down the hamstring when on the ball, and also in the area of your coccyx. This is how you know you've hit pay dirt! Direct pressure works, and so does a little side-to-side motion. Be patient and listen to what your body is telling you, you are your own best therapist!

Gluteus Maximus Mobility

While not really a major contributor to back pain due to trigger points, a tight glute max can hinder our hip mobility, locking up our back and hamstring. Mobilizing the glute max is fairly easy, but also where most people go wrong missing the gluteus minimus and medius completely. No rocket science with this one, here's your model:

Method – Lying on your back, place a lacrosse ball squarely under your glute max and stir the pot moving the ball all over, utilizing your bodyweight for pressure.

Modality – Ideally a lacrosse ball, but you can start with a baseball or softball if your glute is on the sore side.

Time – 4 to 6 minutes of continuous pressure, moving the ball frequently!

Gluteus Maximus Trigger Points

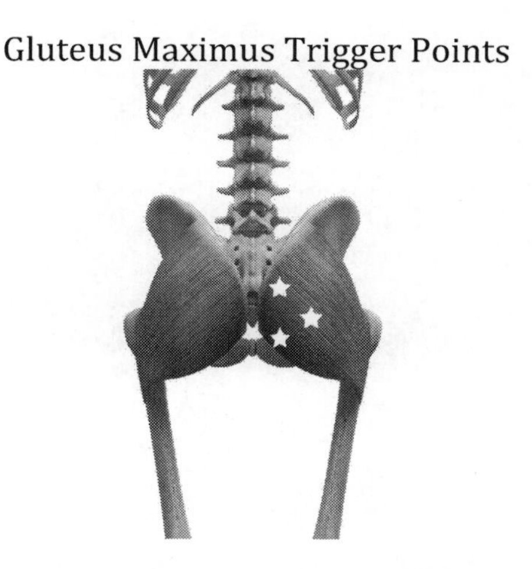

Lying on your back, place the ball in the middle of your glute and roll with both feet on the floor.

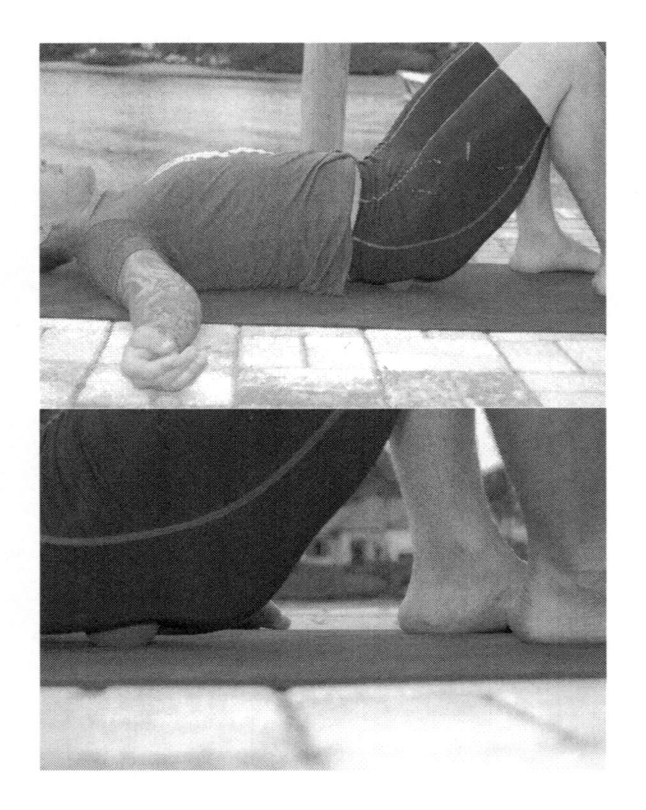

This is one of the easiest mobilizations you will be doing and can often be passed up because of this. Make no mistake; a mobilized glute is much better off than a non-mobilized glute. The pressure will keep the tissue open and free from trigger points caused by excessive sitting and in some cases standing.

Hamstring Mobility

The hamstrings are second in charge to help the lower back do its job. Tight hamstrings create more work and more pressure for the low back muscles and disks to work with. Sitting for prolonged periods of time can easily create trigger points in them, which automatically create a shorter, tighter muscle without us even realizing. Here's your model:

Method – Seated on a counter where the foot can dangle. Place a softball under your thigh and relax your leg. Drag your hamstring on the ball from hip to knee repositioning the ball as necessary. Take note of any bumps, lumps, or hard tissue and focus your efforts in those areas.

Modality – Start off with a softball, then graduate to a baseball when it becomes ineffective.

Time – 4 minutes.

Hamstring trigger points

The Hamstring Group

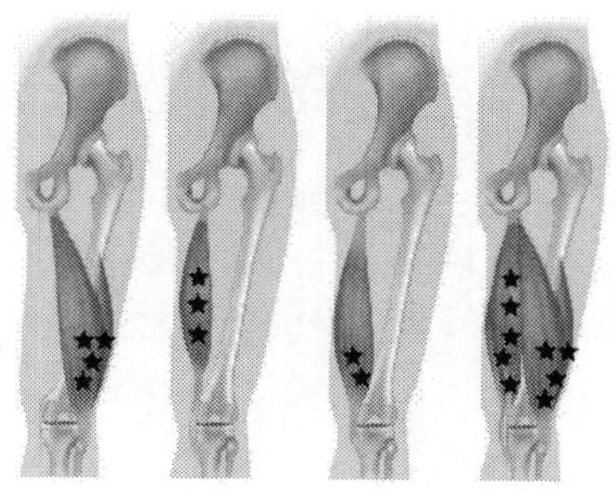

Biceps femoris Semitendinosus Semimembranosus

Sitting on the counter, position the ball under your thigh, directly on your hamstrings.

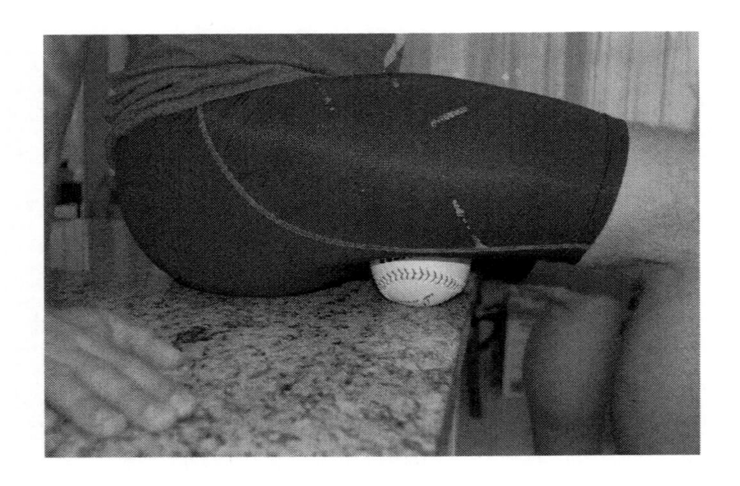

One of the best ways to get more pressure into this mobilization is to introduce movement by extending your lower leg while pinning a tight area down. This is a great way to release adhesions and "unglue" the fascia. Is it still not releasing? Decrease the pressure and increase the frequency at which you extend your leg. Like I said before, mobility is not just about how much pressure you can force on the muscle. The structures underneath (nerves, blood vessels, lymph tracts) are sensitive to pressure as well. Too much pressure and the body may think it is incurring an injury and lock the site down.

Into the mind of the coach: Knowing your "WHY."

With the detail procured to write this book, by now I'm sure you know nothing to this program is random. There is order to everything. Will you get results by going out of order? Sure! However, by going in the order I tell you your results will be *optimized*. Not only are we following the firing patterns for human movement (hip flexors > glutes > hamstrings > low back), but we are also loosening and unlocking the hamstrings before we mobilize them directly. This is because the hamstring tendons emerge from under your gluteal muscles. Tight gluteals will clamp down and shorten your hamstring tendon, tightening the hamstring even though the muscle may not contain any trigger points!

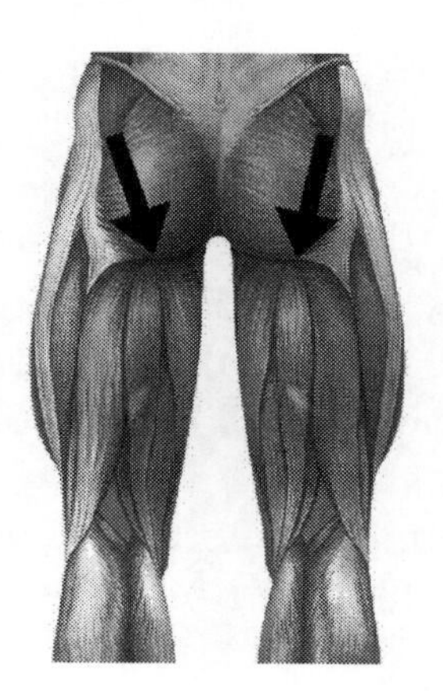

Restoring these damaged, tight structures in order not only sends the right signal to our brain, but also makes the process of returning to health 3-5x easier. Now, let's go see what lies in store for that ailing low back of yours!

Lower Back Mobility

Far from the workhorse, I would more so call your lower back command central. Not that it tells any other muscle group what to do or how to fire, but it commands that they do their part and function correctly or else! Truth be told, we do abuse our lower backs on a daily basis. From the shoes we wear (ladies go above and beyond with their high heels), to the seats we sit in, to the posture we function in, to the way we pick things up without thinking. This is what makes the lower back muscles the workhorse – the sheer abuse they must endure! Your back muscles take very good care of you. They help you move to get to wherever you want to go. When someone comes to me complaining of acute back pain I say, "Your back does a lot for you, what are you doing for your back?" After my weightlifting accident I promised myself I would never entertain back pain again – once was enough. My routine now dictates around 7-10 minutes of daily back mobilization, which allows me to compete at a high level for my age without any back-related pain. This mobilization helps me relax and melt any weightlifting soreness away. Here's your model:

Method – Lying on your back with the roller underneath your hips, start with your hands at your sides and palms down. As you roll up your back to the base of the neck, slowly move your hands overhead at a steady pace. Return down to the hips, moving your arms back to the start position.

Modality – Foam roller.

Time – 8 to 10 minutes.

Start at the base of your spine, hands at your side

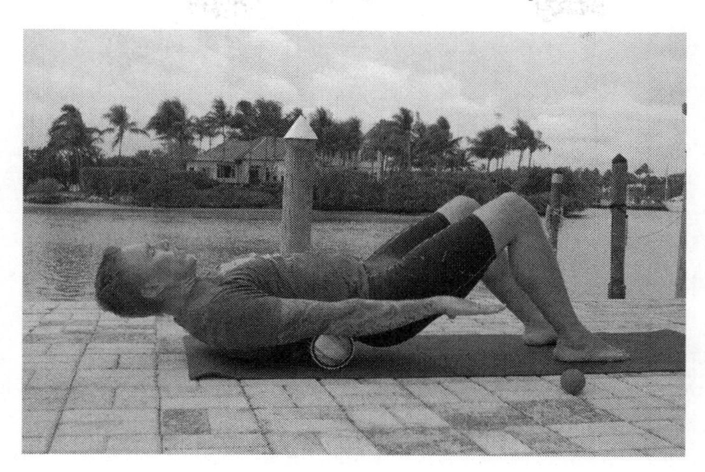

Next, coordinate your arms with the position of the roller

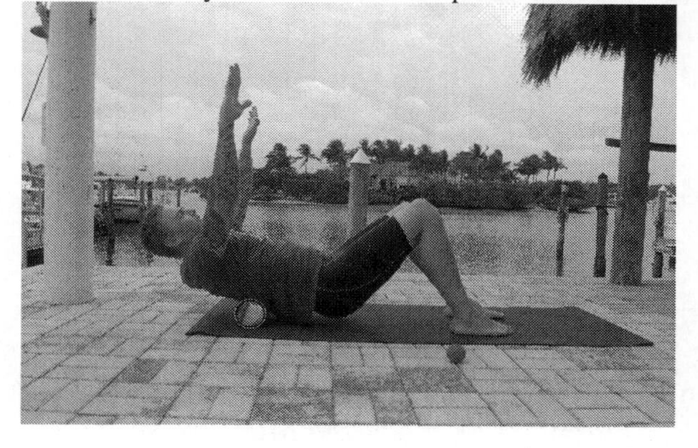

As the roller ends up at the base of your spine, your hands should be in the overhead position.

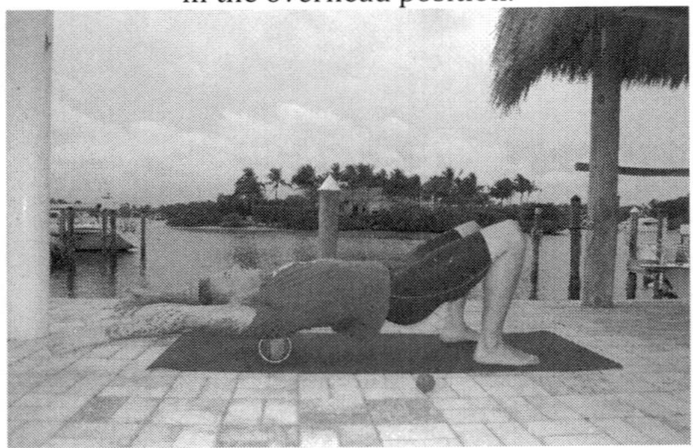

The reason we want to roll the entire back and not just the lower part is because our back is one big sheet of tissue called the thoracolumbar fascia. This layer of fascia attaches to our spine, ribs, pelvis and all of the small and large muscles attached to them, but also has an influence on the abdominal wall. We know pain travels, and as it travels it distorts muscle tissue. You may not have any pain in your middle or upper back, but because it is attached to this fascia, you can be sure there is something brewing in there. This technique is as much preventative as it is restorative and it truly shows the interrelatedness of all of the muscles and its fascia in the trunk of the body. As we said earlier the body is a closed loop; a continuous circle of intertwined tissue penetrating through all things – even bone and organs. It only makes sense that we start with the abdominals, then work the hip flexors, then work the glutes, then work the hamstrings, then work the back, which affects the abdominals again.

When our back is in pain, it's likely that more than one of these muscles is tight, irritated, or containing trigger points. Go through the entire system and check off where you have to work more, where you can work less, and which muscle, or muscles you may not have to work on at all. It's good to stimulate all tissue with pressure from time to time, but if you're hammering away at a glute minimus of yours for 6 minutes and there's no tender areas or pain being referred, it's safe to say that muscle is sound. Work smart, not hard because working smart is working hard!

Pro Tip: Roll out your back before and after the Chiropractor.

Many of the people I have worked with have asked me if I believe in chiropractors, or if they are worth going to. My response is absolutely, as long as you're doing your part as well. What's your part? Foam rolling your back for starters before you go to see the good doctor. Adding the gluteals to that list wouldn't be such a bad idea either.

Vertebrae do not sublux on their own. Poor movement, which leads to muscle spasms, is to blame. What else attaches to the spine but our muscles? Rolling your low back and gluteals before seeing your chiropractor will gently warm the muscles up, loosening the grip they have on subluxed vertebrae making the adjustment more productive and easy. Rolling them after the adjustment helps keep the muscles calm now that the vertebrae are back in their normal place for optimal health.

Ask The Coach: Sitting or Standing Desk?

Best selling author Kelley Starrett puts it plain as day in his new book *Deskbound* when he said, "The typical seated office worker has more musculoskeletal injuries than any other industry sector worker, including construction, metal industry, and transportation workers." The problem exists because the typical office worker does not exert enough physical force on a day to day basis to uncover these musculoskeletal injuries, so they stay hidden for years until chronic pain develops and by that time it is very challenging to reverse said injuries. I'm sure you've heard sitting is the new smoking several times, yet we continue to sit. What's worse is prolonged sitting followed by intense exercise. For some, exercise is an afterthought or done with haste. You sit at work for nearly 8 hours, sit in traffic for an hour on the way home, then jump out of the car, change clothes in a rush, do a stretch or two and then pound the pavement as fast as you can for 20 minutes. Some of you may be saying, "But I don't have time to warm up!" Ask yourself this: Will you have time to heal yourself when an injury strikes?

I'm guessing you won't have time for that either. There are some staggering statistics surrounding the potential sitting has to create disease in the body when there was none. Here are some facts taken from standupkids.org showing what even 2 hours of sitting per day can do:

- Increased risk for Heart Disease
- Increased risk for Diabetes
- Metabolic Syndrome

- Increased risk of Cancer
- Back & Neck Pain

Sitting literally turns your brain, and your body to mush. The posture most of us sit hours with would not be sustainable for even 5 minutes standing, the pain would be too great to bear. A simple search on Amazon will produce a wide variety of standing desk options from $29 all the way up to over $5,000 in some cases. Choose which option is best for you and join your fellow rebel bipeds!

As always, we ask, "What can I do right now?" I've mentioned my 20/20 rule, but it bears repeating here again. Every 20 minutes get up and do something active or athletic for 20 seconds. Be silly and move every joint in a full range of motion. Do Burpees or a cartwheel. Stimulate your muscles and your brain to stop the subsequent decay of both. Your health is in your hands every day, don't take your movement for granted, and realize this precious gift we have all been given and all have the ability to keep if we so choose.

Chapter 6 – Step 2: Stretching

"Body is not stiff, mind is stiff."
-K. Pattabhi Jois

Jessica came to me with some pretty bad low back pain that she said would radiate down into her leg from time to time. When asked about her history, she told me about a horrific car accident she was in 6 years prior. Broken jaw, herniated disks, and contusions – not fun stuff by any means. Refusing to let pain dictate her life, she was still very active. She ran, did yoga, and loved heavy weightlifting. Upon inspection, I noticed right off the bat that her left glute was extremely tight which made a lot of sense because she was hit on her right side. Her left glute was overcompensating during everything she was doing from an activity standpoint and in doing so created a nasty lower crossed syndrome where her left glute tightened up along with her right hip flexor. The left glute muscle was so tight that it was actually creating an impingement in her hip. She was instructed to roll out her left gluteus musculature, as well as her right hip flexor muscle first, and then follow that up with some specific stretches. During her last session she said that her left hip felt like it needed to pop. I told her that it probably did in order to release the muscle fully, open up the hip, and ultimately get rid of the impingement for good. As she inched forward ever so slowly you could see the concern as the pressure built and then a loud pop was heard as her glute finally succumbed to the pressure. She felt a warm sensation flood down her left leg and as she returned to a standing position could not believe the relief she felt in her back. This was only our third session together!

Although she still had some treatment to follow our time together did not last very long after that. Correcting the residual tightness in the hip flexor was now an easy task and the body soon returned to its normal tensegrity. The fact remained that I was treating another crooked set of hips that was creating an ailing lower back. I find this much too often when someone injures a limb on one side of their body, rehabilitates that limb, only to ignore the non-injured limb completely. This is not their fault, but the fault of the rehabilitation specialist. The maxim becomes not only what we do to one side of the body we also do to the other, but instead should be dictated, "What we do to one area of the body can be felt throughout the entire body."

The length of this book whether 200 pages or 2,000 will never be enough for me to reiterate how interconnected our body truly is. Jean-Claude Guimberteau says in his book, *The Architecture of Human Living Fascia,* that our body is a "system of systems." To me, our body is a walking juxtaposition. One strategically placed bullet and we are done for. Yet another person survived from 37 poorly placed stab wounds. Our body can be very fragile at times, yet very resilient at others. When working with our tissue we need to keep this at the forefront of our mind at all times. Jessica didn't force herself into that position to haphazardly explode that muscle, as you will learn in this chapter, stretching is about patiently allowing your body to adjust itself. It's about breathing, repetition, and consistency (Are you willing to stretch those glutes before bed? Or are you too tired and just going to wait till tomorrow?). By now, I think I have sparked your interest enough and it's time to reveal magic step number 2 in my healing process – stretching!

Why We Have to Do It

Stretching always gets the benefit of the doubt, whether it deserves it or not. It is one of the most commonly prescribed things for a tight muscle. The use of foam rollers, lacrosse balls, and softballs for healing the tissue is still under a little bit of an attack though. There are some therapists that criticize self applied massage tools such as foam rollers or lacrosse balls as not being "true" myofascial release and I tend to agree with them. What they are trying to depict is the truest definition of the word "release." They want to claim only a manual therapist can truly "release" a muscle but this is far from true. I along with several other mobility experts have got nothing but amazing results teaching people to be their own best therapist. In my opinion there are 3 major steps to releasing a muscle. Step one was rolling our tissue. If you remember, incorrect muscle firing patterns create tense, fibrotic, and knotted up tissue called trigger points. The pressure provided by our own bodyweight up against the rigidness of the ball or roller will help break up the tissue to decrease the pain response, but it still needs to be unglued and lengthened. This is where stretching comes in. Stretching will help pull apart the glued fascia and help return its ability to glide once again, restoring its original length and allowing the joint it controls to operate in a full range of motion once again.

This is where the incomplete release bit comes from. If you just foam roll, the release is incomplete, but you think you are done because there is no more pain being referred. The tissue may stay glued together and when we return to sport or our regular daily activities the brain still has a hardwire to the damaged area, tightening it right back up, leaving us scratching our head and having to starting back at square one again. Note to self: *just because the pain went away does not mean we are out of the woods yet!* Even though the elimination of the pain is our goal, returning our body to its normal structure and function is always our *mission*. Failing to stretch a muscle after we apply pressure is like winning one battle, and not caring to win the war.

Stretching Rules and Plasticity vs. Elasticity

Stretching is one of those things that everyone knows how to do, right? I mean there's really nothing to it. You're tight, you bend over, the muscles stretch and then you stand back up. I'm sure you know where I'm going with this.... Stretching in this manner is not bad, but it doesn't do very much good for the body either. We are interested in making a permanent change to the tissue, as well as *optimizing* our time while stretching. Stretching haphazardly with no instruction will not lengthen your muscle tissue. This is because muscle is *elastic*, but the fascia that covers the muscle is *plastic*. Let's not forget that the fascia penetrates our muscle tissue all the way down to the bone as well. The bottom line is to make an actual change to what we are stretching; we need to realize we are stretching more than just a muscle.

To get a picture of what I'm talking about, think about a rubber band that is wrapped in a thin coating of plastic. You know the rubber band can expand and contract very quickly and with minimal effort, but what about the plastic? Have you ever tried to break a plastic tag off of a new shirt? Take notice next time how slowly the plastic stretches, and then if it does not break let the tag go and watch how slowly the plastic contracts to regain its original shape and length. This is truly what your muscle tissues do. As a result, my first of several rules to stretching a muscle is always slow going into the stretch and even slower coming out of the stretch. We are stretching the muscle, but if we fail to adhere to the rules of the fascia, we will be stretching for nothing.

There has been a lot of new information on stretching coming out over the last few years. It used to be the only way to warm up until studies found that rigorous stretching actually increased the incidence of injury in sport. This is because when we stretch our muscles and create a change in length, we are disrupting the balance the sensors in our muscles have created. These two sensors are called Golgi tendon organs, and muscle spindle fibers. Golgi tendon organs measure the amount of force (tension) that is being applied to the muscle, and muscle spindle fibers measure the length of the muscle and report this information back to the brain in real time. When we change the length of our muscles through stretching, our brain needs to calibrate the new length-tension agreement before we can do explosive exercise like sprinting, or squatting. Light stretching required a downtime of 15 minutes, and extensive stretching required a downtime of nearly 2.5 hours!

Hopefully you are already getting the idea that stretching is way more than it seems. We have barely scratched the surface though, but for now let's recap on rule #1:

Slow going in, slower coming out.

My second rule to stretching is to breathe correctly. Wow, here we go with the breathing thing again! Have you ever had a friend help you with a stretch and accidently push you too far? Did you ever take note of what happened? I'm betting your ability to breathe got cut off. This is because we have a negative feedback loop in our body that relates our ability to stretch with our ability to breathe. Think about it, if you are stretching a muscle to far too fast where you can potentially injure yourself, what would be a quick response your body could produce to stop you from doing that? Breathing, that's what! Our yogi friends have it right when they are promoting the breath while stretching and this is where many people fail when trying to make a change in flexibility.

To stretch properly, our breath must be under a constant state of control. We inhale before the stretch and then exhale through the stretch. This turns off that negative feedback loop in the brain and allows us to take control of what limits stretching the muscle, rather than the mind controlling the limits of the stretch. Never hold your breath or suffocate yourself during stretching. Controlling the normalcy of your breath will keep the nerves calm and allow you to achieve a deeper, more permanent stretch.

Rule #2:

Inhale before the stretch, exhale during the stretch.

Rule number three is already systematically built into the program, but is worth noting and explaining into greater detail and that is always roll before you stretch! I have said it before; putting pressure on your muscles sends a message back to the brain for that area to relax. If we are lucky enough to get that area of tissue to actually release, then the stretch will help open it to a much greater extent. I actually found this out the hard way when I was training for a marathon in Honolulu one year. With all of the running and weightlifting I was doing, my hamstrings started to tighten up on me considerably, producing discomfort in both my lower back and calf muscles. A friend of mine was a bikram yoga instructor and told me a class or two would clear me right up. She invited me to partake and I wasted no time in trying to open these suckers up. While the stretching was intense and my flexibility did improve, the pain actually got worse in my calf muscles. I found out later this was due to the tightening of the trigger points in my hamstrings. In Clair Davies' wonderful book *The Trigger Point Therapy Workbook*, he cautions against stretching before applying pressure due to the tightening effect it can have on active trigger points. Unfortunately, I didn't have this information available to me at the time, but you certainly do! So rule #3 is:

Always apply pressure before stretching!

Rule #4 is an interesting one, and that's to stretch actively, and not passively. My definition for this is to always be moving, especially for some of our deep hip stretches. To do this, we can provide a little bounce, a wave motion, or a circular motion. The key is to do this very gently. There's a huge difference between stretching a muscle and stretching a joint capsule, especially one like the hip. Pinning yourself down in a hamstring stretch and creating a lot of pain is never a good idea. Remember, movement heals, isolation and immobilization prolong healing. While some of our stretches may seems like we are isolating a muscle, really each stretch is designed to open up the hip capsule by also stretching some of the surrounding musculature at the same time.

Rule #4:

Stretch actively, not passively.

The first time I heard about this way of stretching was in 2006 through a book called *Stretch to Win* written by Chris and Ann Frederick. They had a simple concept they were trying to introduce – stretch the fascia and win! As soon as I started to institute this concept with my athletes and myself we were achieving new ranges of motion almost instantly.

Two Tests

I love learning about anything related to the human body, especially when it comes to movement or pain free movement. I research new ways of improving mobility constantly, and always ask my clients some of the good things they have taken from people or procedures that have not worked for them in the past. If I find a technique I have never heard of before or one I feel needs further explanation of how to do it, I will visit the practitioner and pay for a treatment. I've been poked, prodded, hooked up to machines, and assessed for up to 30 minutes before any type of treatment was done.

Sometimes the therapist/practitioner comes to a correct conclusion, and other times they are way off the mark. In my opinion, the eye should be the first assessment. I can sometimes tell a client what their problem is before they even open their mouth. Other times I will have them perform one of two tests, which take literally 15 seconds from beginning to end. The first is the hip impingement test, which is where I experienced my first pop in my tissue just like Jessica. Chris and Ann Frederick (*Stretch to Win*) had a simple test for hip impingement, which is where the muscles surrounding a nerve get so tight that they actually get suffocated, creating pain and numbness in the area. I did the test for my right leg and had no problem. When performing the test on my left leg I found I had a real big problem. The test was simple. Lay on your back with one leg straight. Pull the other knee into your chest as much as possible and see if there is a pinching sensation that originates in your hip.

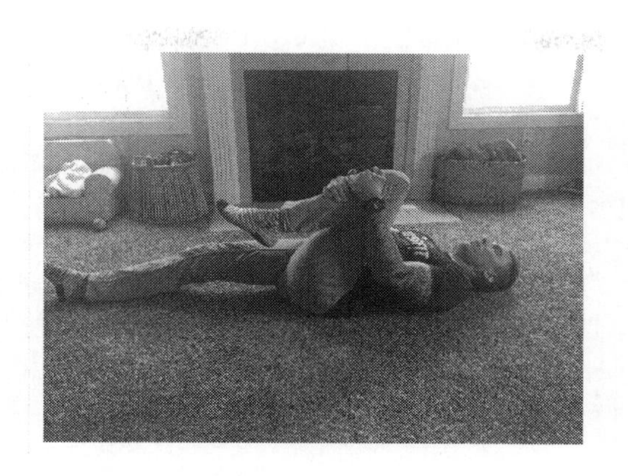

As I applied the principles I learned in the book about active stretching, and stretching fascia not muscles, I was sitting in front of the TV one day stretching my left glute and heard a loud pop in my hip feeling a warm rush of blood down my leg shortly after. It took some time for me to achieve this, as I'm sure it will take you, but like everything else we talk about in this book we must apply the Kaizen principle to stretching as well. With some stretches you may see an instant increase in mobility and flexibility. In other instances, it may take a few months in order to get where you want. Avoid our human tendency to think more is more. Don't force yourself into positions your body is not ready for, snapping out of them like a wound up rubber band. Approach every day as if it's your first day, be gentle, be consistent, and the results will come—trust me!

My second test is the glute stretch test. This test is simple as well and we are trying to find any type of unilateral tightness that has developed through our many years of movement on this Earth. The first thing you want to do is to find something you can put your foot on that is knee height. Place one foot on the object, then whichever foot is on the floor, take a little bit of a step back to put your glute/hamstring complex on a little bit of a pre-stretch. Next we ideally would like to bend forward at the hip only keeping the back neutral. I find however that it makes no difference if you round your back or keep it straight, if you have one glute tighter than the other, you will definitely be able to tell either way. Do this stretch on both sides and see which side allows you to bend lower – this is the loose side.

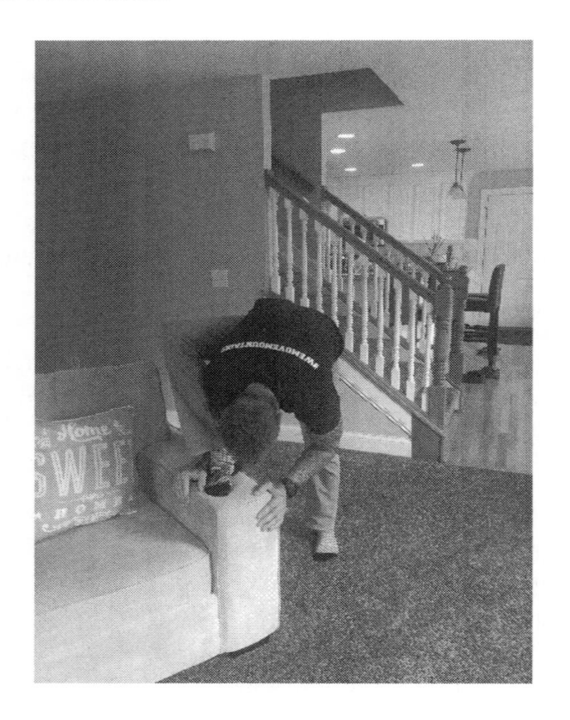

Have a friend, family member, or roommate take a picture of you so you can get a clear idea of how tight you actually are and the urgency needed in the matter.

Pictures work wonders for some clients who have a decreased sense of body awareness. I have shown some clients their unilateral differences much to their disbelief. Their pain and discomfort then makes that much more sense to them! Even though we have so much more to learn, I really truly hope you are not feeling overwhelmed yet and are starting to realize how easy all of this is. I hope my words are providing a sense of calm for you and there is a picture starting to develop in your head of exactly what is wrong, and every page is another brick in the road of where you have to go. Having said that, I can already read your mind – bring on the stretches!

The Modified Lunge

This stretch is a compliment to the glute test I just spoke about. If you are very tight, this is a great way to get started; hence, that is why this is our first stretch in the series. For this stretch we start in a finished lunge position. The forward foot is on the floor, with the opposite knee on the floor, foot pointing behind you.

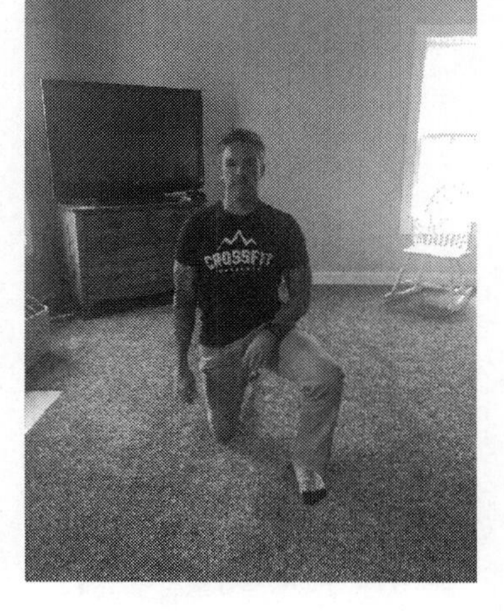

From here, bend forward at the hips allowing for a slight (let me reiterate slight) bend in the lower back. Wrap your hand down on the outside of your foot, and if you can, place your palm firmly on the ground.

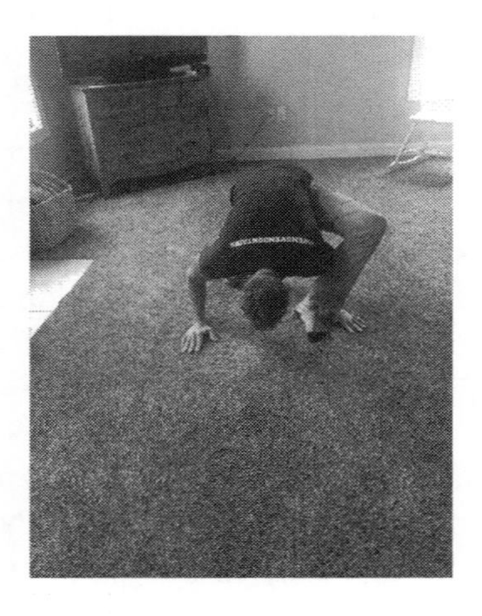

If you cannot put your palm on the ground, place a thick book next to your foot and try to get your palm flat on the book.

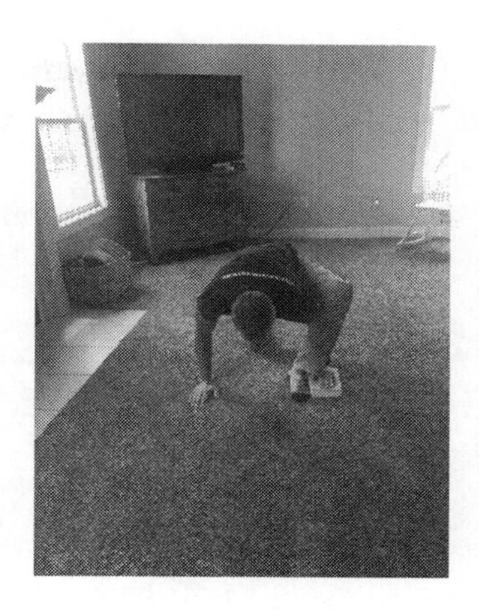

Our goal here is to eventually reach our forehead to the ground as I show below.

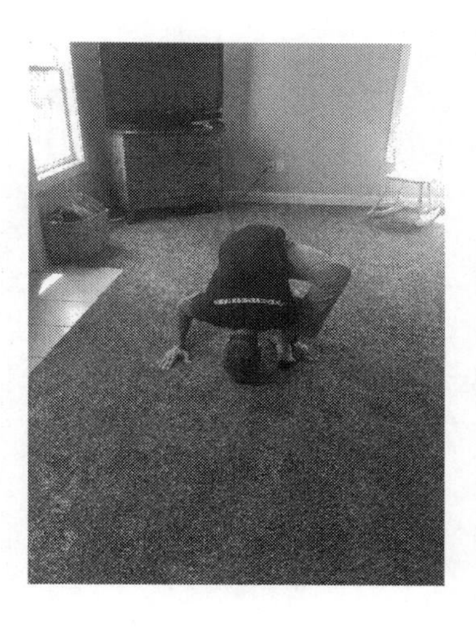

We can perform this stretch with a slight back and forth rocking motion, making sure to exhale every time we stretch if you are really tight. For those who have a little bit more flexibility we want to wave stretch, which means taking a nice deep breath at the top and then exhaling as we descend into the stretch. When we can go no further into the stretch we return to the starting position, inhaling as we come back up, then returning back down into the stretch as we exhale, trying to get down a little further.

Set a timer and perform this stretch for 2 minutes continuously starting with your tighter side. My rule for stretching is 2 to 1 tight side to loose. If your right glute is tighter, stretch the right first, then the left side, then go back and stretch the right side one more time. In the case of a severe one-sided tightness I will have my clients only stretch the tight side, after rolling their tissue of course!

The Couch Pose Stretch

I adopted this stretch from the first yoga class I ever went to – it is originally called a tree pose. The tree pose is supposed to help improve focus, and calm your mind. If you can do a fully knee bent tree pose, chances are you are not reading this book. If you are reading this book then we are going to start off with the couch pose, and hopefully one day achieve just a standing tree pose.

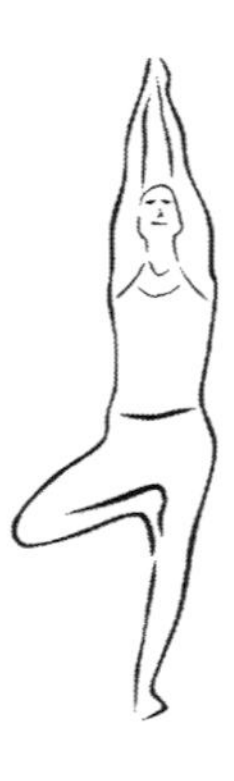

This stretch is one of my favorite ways to target and stretch the glute medius. The higher the back of your couch, the more challenging this stretch will be, but the more you will feel it in your gluteus medius. As always, start off slowly, let gravity help you rest into the stretch and avoid the temptation to grab the couch to wrench yourself into a deeper position.

Start off behind the couch like so, pulling the couch away from the wall if need be.

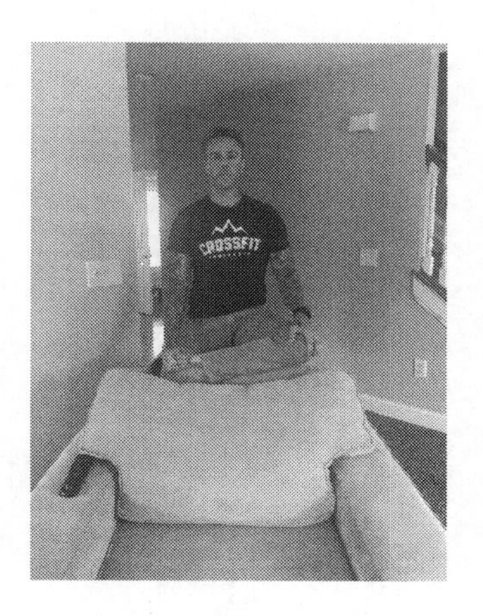

Place your leg up on the back of the couch, ideally with the entire side of your leg resting on the couch. If you can't do this, don't worry; your knee can be up a bit and you can still do the stretch properly. From there we take a deep breath in and exhale as we bend forward at the hip. Same rules apply, you can have a slight bend forward of the back, just make sure you are not bending so much that you are going into C-spine.

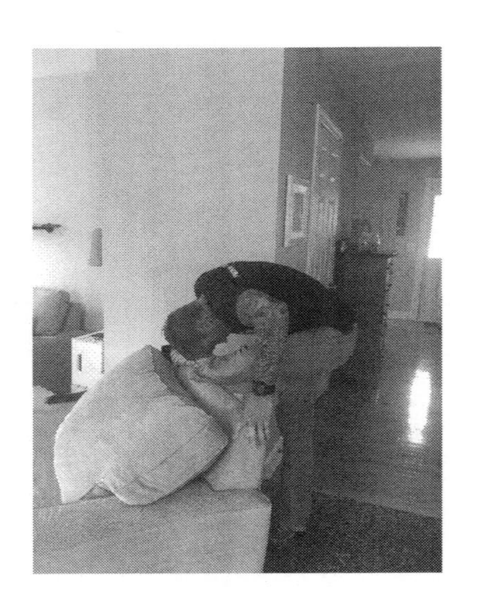

This is an ideal position:

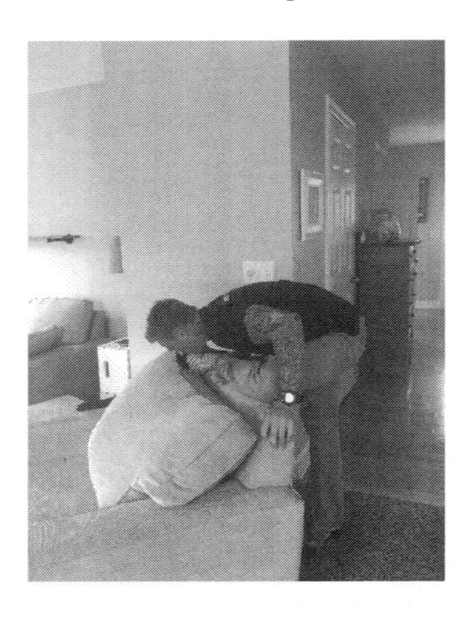

We can start off trying to get our head down to our shin at first, and when our flexibility improves we can switch gears and start to make the destination our foot.

Because of the advanced nature of this stretch it is best to take it slow once again. If you can not even get your foot up on the back of your couch, then I would suggest staying with the modified lunge until you can achieve a forehead to ground position first. Performing the couch pose after will be a nice compliment to continue opening up your gluteus medius. Perform this stretch in a wave pattern, taking a nice deep breath inhalation at the top and then exhaling as you descend down to your shin/foot. Set the time for 2 minutes and relax into the stretch, utilizing our 2 to 1 ratio stretching the tight side to the loose side.

The 75 – 90 – 120 Stretch

This stretch has three parts to it and really packs a wallop towards the end. This is a great example of how we stretch a joint rather than just a muscle. To start, we want to sit on the floor with one leg behind us at the 90-degree position, and the other leg in front of us in the 75-degree position.

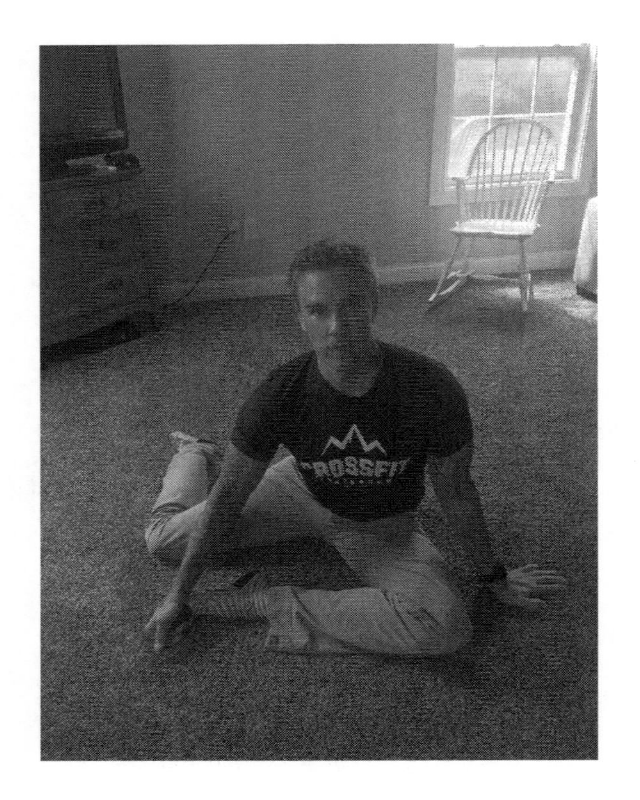

From here we want to take a nice deep breath in and exhale as we bend forward at the hip bringing our head towards, and as close to our foot as possible. Work the tissue in a wave pattern for two minutes allowing gravity to help you relax into the stretch.

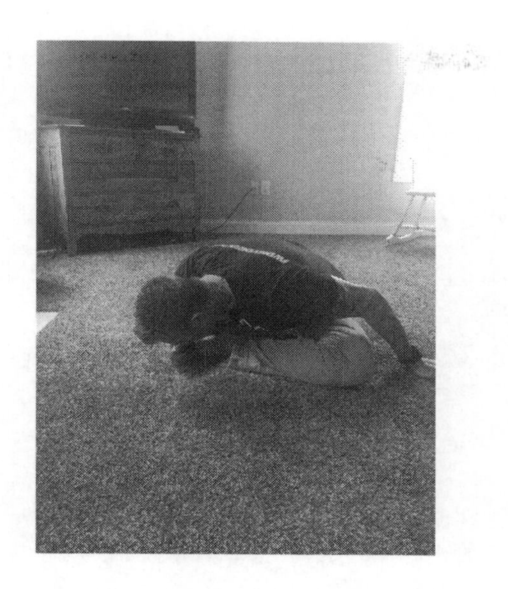

Our next position is to kick our front foot out so we have both legs at 90 degrees. This one is going to be a little harder now.

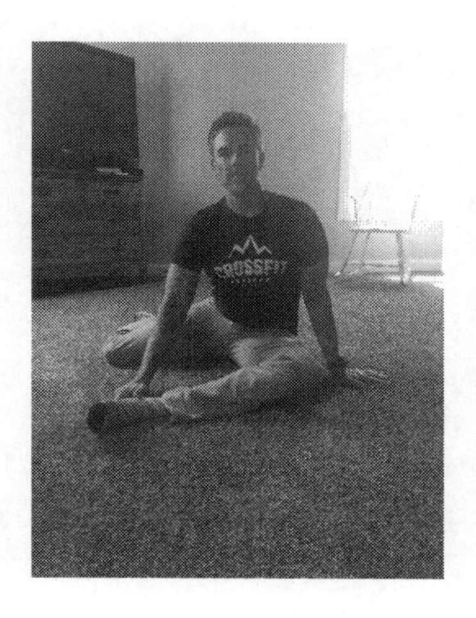

Repeat the same wave pattern trying to get your forehead down to your foot. Set your timer for 2 minutes again and exhale every time you relax down into that stretch.

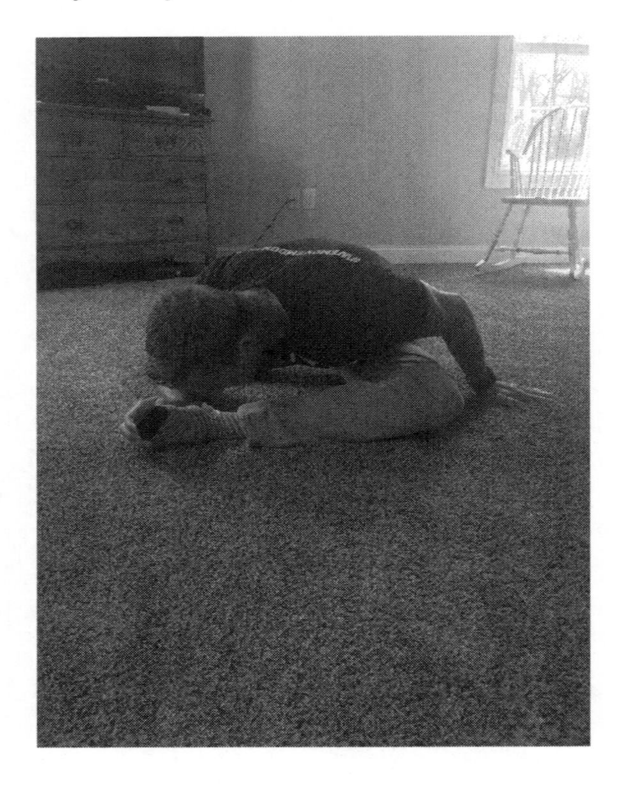

Our last stretch is the kicker and some of you may be so tight that you cannot even achieve a stretch in this position. If this is the case, only perform the first two stretches at 75 and 90 degrees until you gain flexibility and are able to get this one right. To perform this stretch, move your foot out even further so it is at 120 degrees.

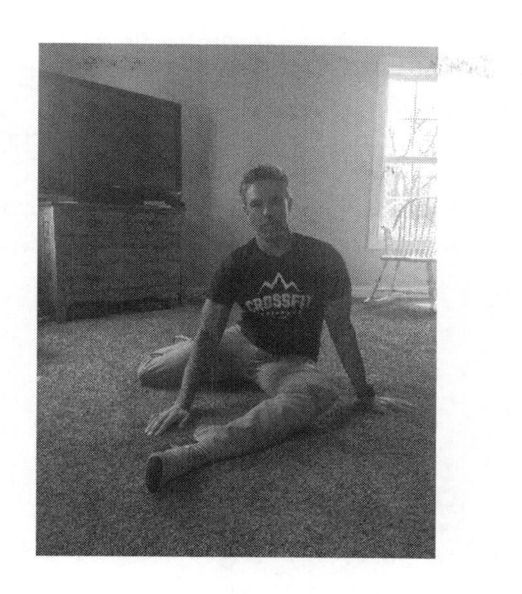

Take a nice deep breath in and exhale as you slowly descend down as low as possible.

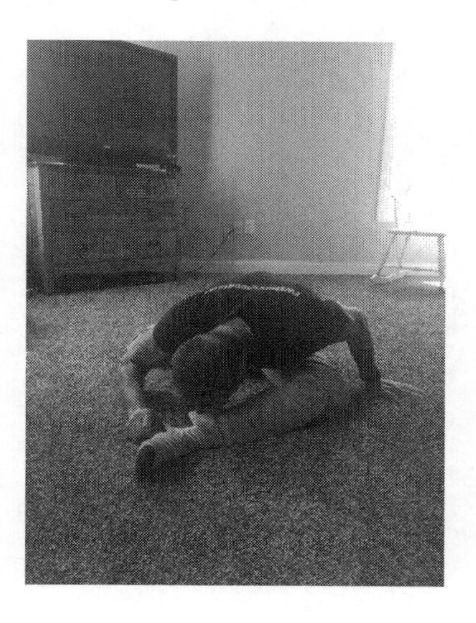

Set your clock for two minutes and develop a nice slow rhythm as you work at unlocking the tissue surrounding your hip joint. For those of your who are looking to accelerate your progress we can add a side-to-side movement I call the pendulum. This pendulum movement will really break up the surrounding fascia and help open up the joint even more.

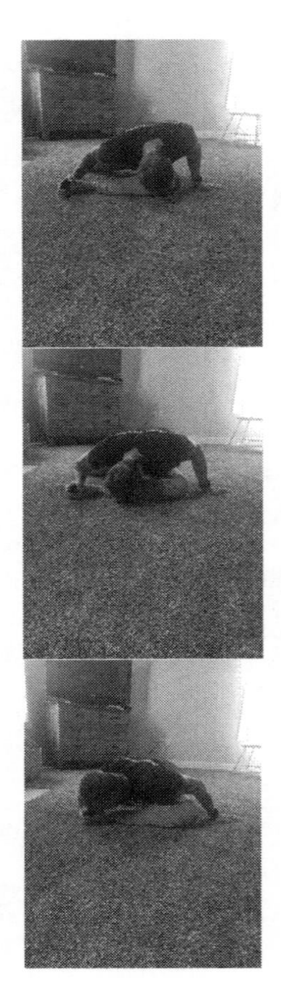

When you complete all three positions for 2 minutes each, we then want to switch legs starting the process all over again with the 75-degree leg position. I realize this is a long one, but it is also a very effective one so the same rules still apply. Stretch the tight side first for 6 minutes, then the loose side for 6 minutes, then back to the tight side for a final 6 minutes. To some, this may seem excessive, but a paltry 18 minutes of stretching pales in comparison to the destruction your normal, every-day movement, posture, and positions have created. The pain you are experiencing at this point is a process of priorities, or a lack of them per se. Has health really been a priority to you? If not, it is time you start to make it a priority. This book, the mobility exercises in the previous chapter and these stretches are a great start. Like we said earlier, awareness is the first key. Being aware of every movement, no matter how big or small, is our first key to feeling better.

The Hip Flexor Stretch with Rotation

If you thought our last 75-90-120 stretch was starting to get complicated, welcome to the hip flexor stretch with rotation. When executed correctly, there is no better stretch to open your hips up and make you feel like a spring chicken again. For those of you who run, or love fire breathing through CrossFit, Tough Mudders, or Spartan races you will notice that after doing this stretch your breathing will become less laborious and it may even feel like you have an extra lung. This is because the fascia of your hip flexors is connected to the fascia of your diaphragm, and the fascia of your diaphragm is connected to the fascia of your heart. Funny how the body does that huh? The prime muscle used in forward movement is connected to what helps us breathe and circulate blood. You can do this stretch in one of two ways either on the floor or on a couch – it just depends which one you are more comfortable on. To understand completely what this stretch offers we must get a little bit into what the hip flexors actually do, because to stretch them we are going to undo what it does. Yes, that's how funky your hip flexors are!

The first action your hip flexors perform that we are going to talk about is lateral flexion meaning your right hip flexor helps you bend to the right. So if we are stretching the right hip flexor, how do we undo what it does? We tilt our upper body to the left!
The second motion your hip flexors contribute to is rotation to the opposite side of your body. So staying with the right hip flexor, this means it will also rotate your upper body to the left, which means during this stretch, we will be rotating to face right.

The third job your hip flexors have is to extend your lumbar vertebrae which makes you look like you have a belly out position. To undo this action, we tuck our tail and posteriorly rotate our pelvis by pulling up on our lower abdominals (please don't fall asleep yet, this is just getting good!).

Fourth, the hip flexors flex the hip! So to undo this we are going to extend the hip.
Fifth, the hip flexors externally rotate the thigh bone, so part of this stretch is going to include us internally

rotating the thigh bone which will rotate our foot out away from us.
All too often I see people getting into a tremendously grotesque position to chase a hip flexor stretch. Their back has a huge arch, their head is extended backwards and it looks like they are trying to bend in half backwards at the hip. This will all too often reinforce its tightness. To stretch the intricacies of this muscle we need to develop a very robust position while trying not to yield to its uncomfortable nature. The following guide is the best and most stable way I have found to get into the stretch and don't worry, getting out of it is much, much easier.

First we are going to start in the modified lunge position again.

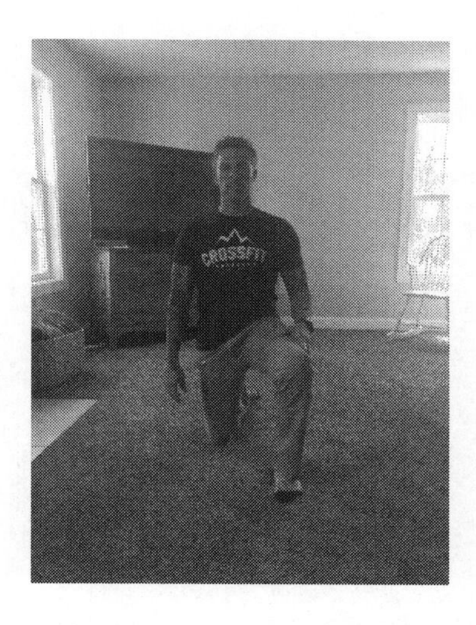

From here keeping our spine neutral, we are going to internally rotate our femur, which will externally rotate our foot moving it further away from the midline of our body.

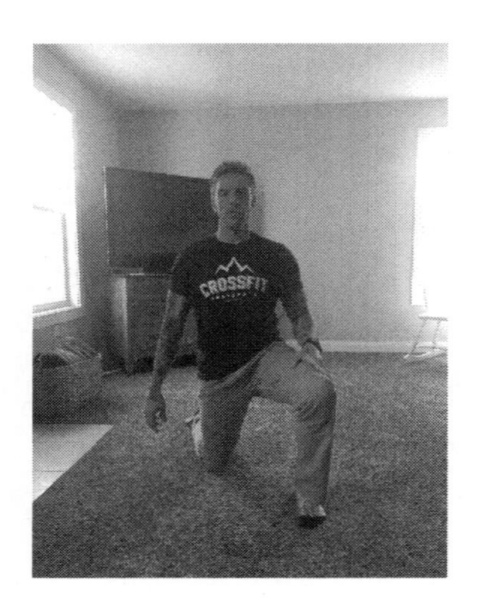

Next, we want to bring the opposite leg close to our knee making it look like we are trying to kneel on a tight rope.

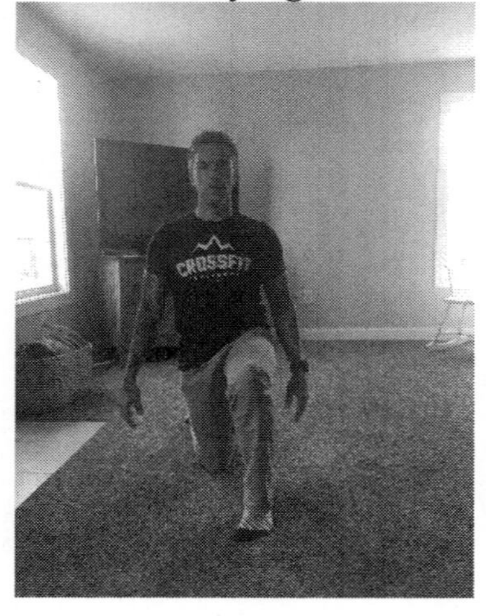

Fourth, we want to tuck our tail by pulling up on our lower abdominal muscles, not by just squeezing our gluteal muscles. This takes some getting used to, be patient and get it right as the pay off is a big one. This gets the hip flexor out of its lumbar flexion component and usually when you get it right will produce an instant stretch in the front of your hip.

Tail Not Tucked

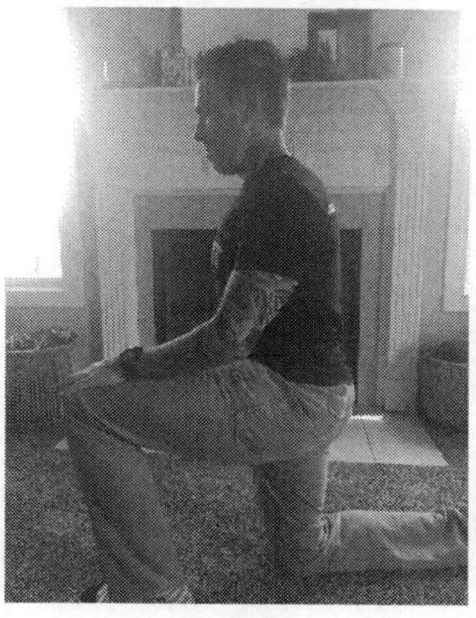

Tail Tucked (Notice the flatness of my lower back)

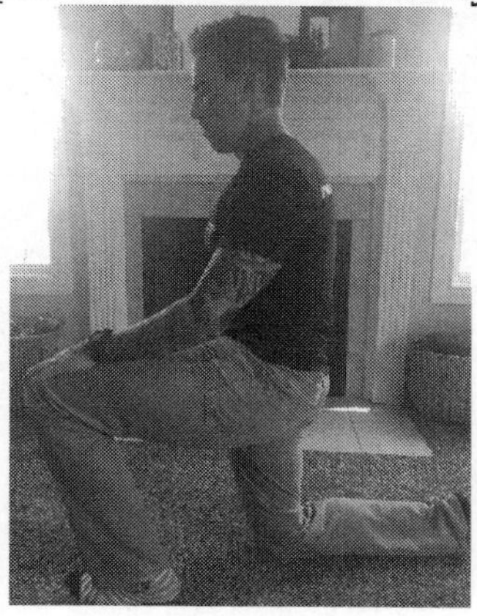

Now that I have you all off balance and ready to tip over from a stiff breeze, we want to side bend slightly away from the side that we are stretching, which will loosen up our lateral flexion component.

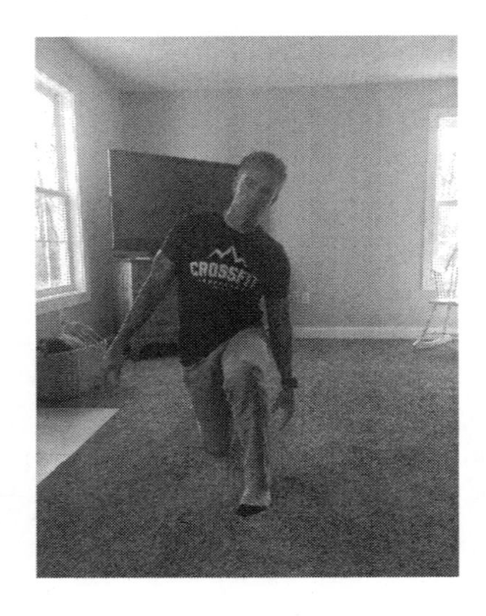

Our last movement to undo what the hip flexor does in order to stretch it correctly is to rotate to the side we are trying to stretch. Also, we want to extend the arms in front, externally rotate our hands with the fingers spread wide and pull our wrists back, this is a full fascial stretch. Remember we are not in the business of isolating a single muscle!

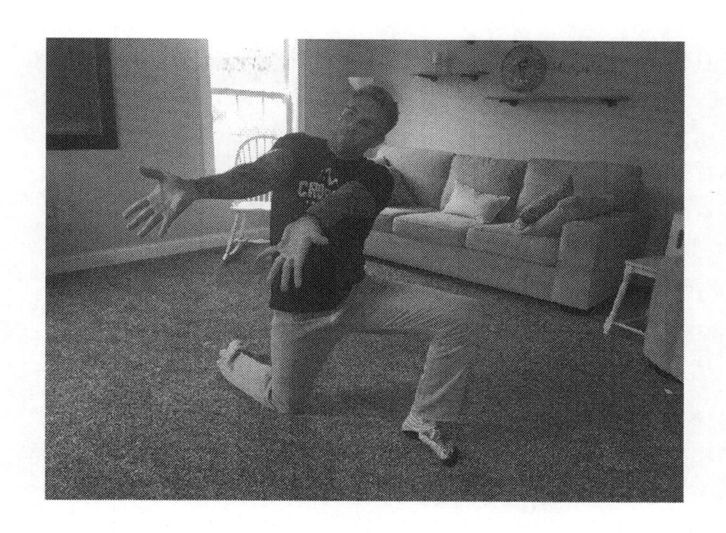

Once we complete the final step to this stretch we want to stay in the stretch for one minute. Remember to take a deep breath in before going into the final part of the stretch and then exhale as you begin to rotate. Once you have reached the extent of your ability to rotate you can then practice normal box breathing inhaling for a four count and then exhaling for a four count.

Getting out of the stretch is simple, but remember: it must be done slowly. When your minute is up, slowly rotate back to facing forward, and then to finish off and come out of the stretch lean forward taking the pressure of the stretch off of your hip flexors. Switch legs and repeat the step-by-step process we just discussed.

Coach's Tip! Are you having difficulty discerning which hip flexor is tight for our 2 to 1 rule? As consistent as death and taxes, the glute that is tight will naturally produce a tight opposite hip flexor. This means if your left glute tested as the tight one, then your right hip flexor will be tight as well. Sometimes it's too slight to feel, and other times it is blatantly obvious. Do your due diligence and give that tight one some extra love!

The Van Damme Stretch

I grew up watching Sylvester Stallone movies, Arnold Schwarzenegger movies, and especially Jean-Claude Van Damme movies. I loved Stallone for his toughness, Arnold for his physique, and Van Damme for his athleticism and martial arts. I was enamored by the positions Van Damme put his body in and wanted to achieve the splits he performed in the movies so one day I took two boxes and spread them apart, put a foot on each one and tried to "ease" into a split. I'm sure I don't have to tell you this did not go well. Stepping back 30,000 feet and assessing the situation, I realized if I put a prop in the middle I could support myself and then put the "ease" back in easy. In doing so I proceeded to get the best adductor, hamstring, and gluteus minimus stretch I've ever had in my life. Cleverly, I nicknamed these "Van Dammes."

You'll be happy to know that in order for you to get the same benefit out of the Van Damme stretch you will not have to prop yourself up and balance like a tripod. You, sir or madam, will remain safely grounded. This doesn't mean that I'm taking it easy on you though. To effectively do the Van Damme stretch for your hamstring/groin/glute complex, you need to start with your feet spread as wide as possible while internally rotating your feet at the hip.

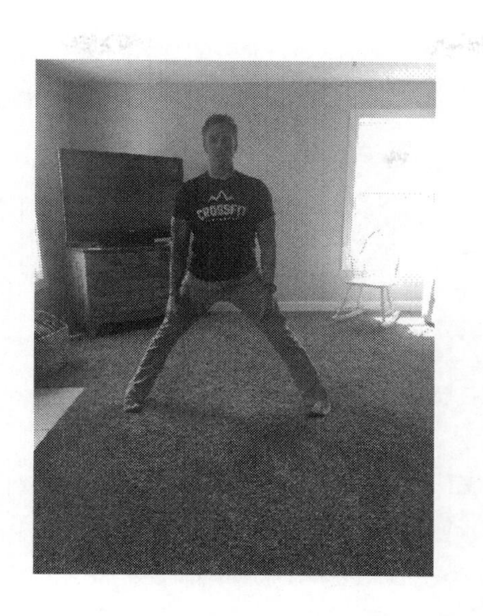

From here, your next step is to bend over and put your palms flat on the floor pushing your butt back.

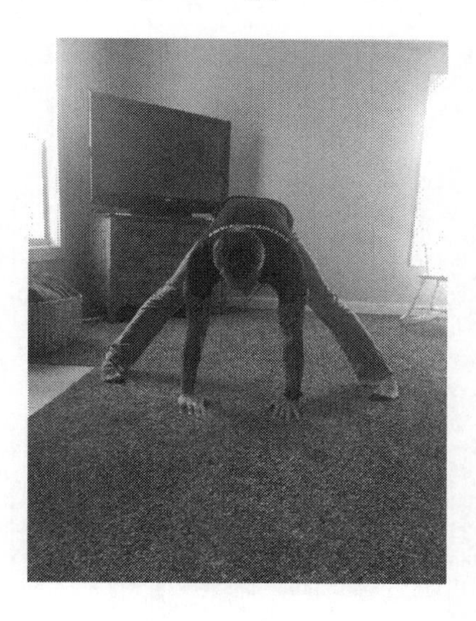

If this position is too easy for you, your next step is to put your elbows on the floor.

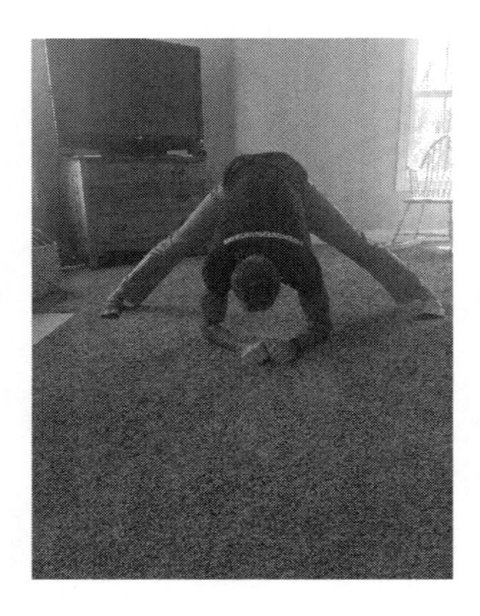

If you can put your elbows on the floor with no problem, then the last step is to get your forehead to touch the ground.

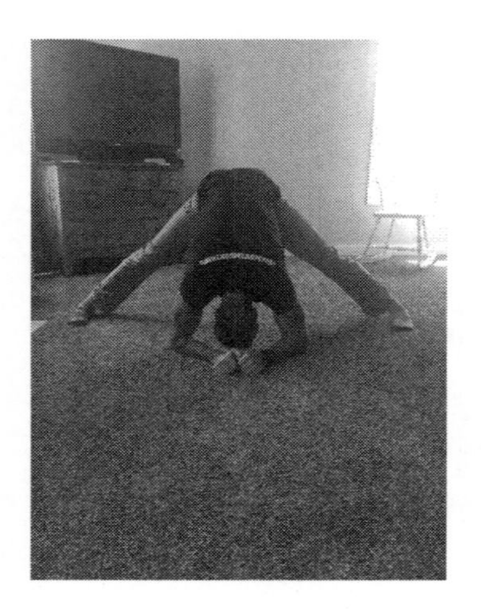

You can literally keep progressing this stretch until you obtain a split. You can keep spacing your feet apart, and keep relaxing into the stretch further and further until you get closer and closer to the floor. This stretch is going to be held for two minutes, which at first seems to be closer to 5 minutes. Remember to exhale as you descend into your initial stretch, and then as gravity does its thing, focus on your box breath of four seconds on the inhale and four seconds on the exhale. When you're finished, slowly inch your feet back together, pausing for a few seconds after each step if you wish. We don't want to collapse or snap out of the stretch as we've discussed returning our beautiful fascia to back to how it was with no change essentially wasting that two minutes we spent in what is sometimes agony. I know coming out of these stretches sometimes is difficult, but it's not as difficult as having to do it all over again because of a sloppy exit.

Like I said earlier, stretching always gets the benefit of the doubt in any situation and is as revered as breathing. It's commonplace to see a runner stretching on a park bench and not think anything about it. He or she is warming up as they should, but sadly they are not making the change that they think. There have been many studies published about the efficacy of static stretching and the results have been poor at best. Just look at a few of the studies conducted:

1. Konrad A, Tilp M. Increased range of motion after static stretching is not due to changes in muscle and tendon structures. *Clin Biomech (Bristol, Avon)*. 2014 May 9. (Many people think stretching

increases the muscles length, clearly by the title we are finding otherwise.)

2. Shrier I. Stretching before exercise does not reduce the risk of local muscle injury: a critical review of the clinical and basic science literature. *Clin J Sport Med.* 1999;9. (People think stretching before exercise reduces injury, and it clearly does not.)
3. Kay AD, Blazevich AJ. Effect of Acute Static Stretch on Maximal Muscle Performance: A Systematic Review. *Med Sci Sports Exerc.* 2011 Jun 8. (Researchers looked at data from 4,500 studies on stretching and found overwhelming evidence of no significant effect for performance; hence, stretching does not make you a better athlete.)
4. Lund H. The effect of passive stretching on delayed onset muscle soreness, and other detrimental effects following eccentric exercise. *Scand J Med Sci Sports.* 1998 Aug;8(4):216–21. (There was no difference seen between the control and experimental groups, so stretching does not take away soreness either.)
5. Ylinen J, Kautiainen H, Wiren K, Hakkinen A. Stretching exercises vs manual therapy in treatment of chronic neck pain: a randomized, controlled cross-over trial. *J Rehabil Med.* 2007;39(2):126–132. (People think stretching reduces pain. This trial of 125 patients found pretty promising benefits to both stretching exercises and "manual therapy" for a month, and the researchers concluded that "low-cost stretching exercises can be recommended in the first instance as an appropriate therapy

intervention to relieve pain, at least in the short-term."—Wait, what???)

There it was! I'm sure you were wondering why I was recommending stretching exercises, and then telling you stretching doesn't do anything. Well, it turns out that stretching may really only be good for one thing – people with pain who are also combining it with manual therapy! That's what we are doing here, ladies and gents. People with pain as we have already depicted have created an environment in their body that is producing a constant state of contraction even when you are at rest. This constant contraction draws the muscle into a shortened state making it tight, and reducing our mobility. The main reason we stretch in this program is not to increase the length of our musculature; it is to return the length to normal! Ultimately yes, we are increasing the length of the muscles, and the fascia, but we are not taking the muscle from its normal length to a longer length, we are taking the muscle from a shortened contracted length to a normal length.

Your Keys to Success

1. Always roll the fascia before you stretch.
2. Realize you are returning the fascia, and muscle to its normal resting length and no further.
3. We are increasing the range of motion of the joint as well.
4. Inhale before stretching, exhale during.
5. Slow going in, slow coming out.

Ask the Coach: Should I Go See a Massage Therapist?

The short answer here is yes, absolutely. The long answer is a bit, well, longer. There are so many different manual therapists out there, and because massage therapy isn't cheap it's challenging to find someone who not only understands your condition, but also can provide a solid road map for you to return to health. A general massage, or "feel good" massage as I like to call them, is not targeted enough to make a change to the state of the tissue, nor are they addressing the problem. Rather, these sessions are designed to stimulate endorphins and provide total body relaxation. I've had many clients tell me they were so relaxed they fell asleep during the session. Good luck doing that with me! Like I have stated before, pain is never the purpose of what we do, it is simply part of the process.

Sports massages may be a little more targeted, but still fail to correct the actual problem. The pressure may be a little bit more intense, but if your feet hurt, I find the therapist targeting the feet when there are plenty of trigger points in the calf muscle and hamstring that refer pain into the foot. Once again we are missing the mark. Shiatsu massages are much more intense, primarily using elbows and knees to stimulate blood flow and lymph drainage. They have been known to decrease pain from time to time, but still are not an optimal form of body treatment because it fails to target where the problem is specifically coming from.

Even though there are several types of massage left (lomi-lomi, hot stone, deep tissue, Thai, reflexology) they all still fail at one main (and very important) point: they're all treating symptoms, not the actual problem. So what to do then? Be specific and let your fingers do the walking. Call therapists up and ask them if they have heard of Erik Dalton, Paul Kelly, or if they know how to do fascial stretching. Ask them if they have ever heard of Jean-Claude Guimberteau, or Guy Voyer (Voy-ay [they're both French]). Ask them if they are familiar with trigger points, and if they have read anything from Clair Davies. Any hesitation on their part should constitute caution on yours.

Your other option is to work with me. Yes, that's right, I work with people all over the nation, even though my home base is in South Florida. If you're interested in working with me shoot me an e-mail at chris@influentialhealthsolutions.com even if you just want to say hi and ask a quick question. I love getting to know my readers and it gives me the chance to thank you for your support in believing what I do. As a quick reminder, you can also access the video course with 10x more information and a full 3 month program for a small fee by emailing me as well.

Chapter 7 – Step 3: Motility

"The world breaks everyone, and afterward some are strong at the broken places."
–Ernest Hemingway, A Farewell to Arms

Adam woke up in the middle of the night thinking the house was on fire. He looked down at his leg where he felt the heat (blowtorch is the word he used) and touch it to try to figure out was going on. The pain was ridiculously intense so he tried to stand up and walk around, but as he tried to apply pressure to his right leg it wouldn't respond. Now he was concerned. He tried extending and flexing his leg—although painful, he was still able to move. As he tried to stand up his back started to throb tremendously. Adam was a strong dude and was not a stranger to pain. He played outside linebacker for a major division one college, but at 38 years of age now he worked harder at his day job than he did on his body. More accurately, he was sitting more now than he ever had in his entire life.

Adam came to see me he was concerned to say the least, and so was I. I asked him about injuries, but he couldn't remember anything that would cause such severe pain. As we started to assess him and talk about his life he told me he recently took a job nearly 40 miles further than his previous job because of better pay, hours, and benefits. He also bought a new car as well. Through his assessment we started to uncover a serious tightness he developed in his right low back, right glute, and right hamstring. He reiterated again that he never had an injury on that side. I then asked him to lie on his back on the floor so I could check the length of his legs to see if there was a disparity. As he lay down he made a noise as if he was in pain, and to my amazement he said, "Sorry, I just laid down on my wallet." He proceeded to take the wallet out of his back right side pocket. It was then that alarm bells went off!

I proceeded to ask Adam if he always kept his wallet in his back pocket and he said yes. What we found out was Adam's new car had smaller bucket seats than he was used too. He loved the car, but constantly felt cramped. With the increase in his drive time every day, and an increase in sitting during the day at his job, Adam was literally sitting crooked for hours on end. Because he is such a big guy, rather than the pain developing slowly, his body literally sustained a crooked pelvis for as long as it could until one day the compression became too great and he was awakened in the middle of the night. Mobility work around the hip and back loosened the structures to decrease the pain, and then he was prescribed the proper stretching exercises to return the tissue to its original length. But there was another problem. After we corrected his pelvis he said his leg felt wobbly and weak so I then prescribed some single and double leg exercises, which provided a neuromuscular "Reboot" so to say. Being a college athlete his body learned very quickly and he was pain free in close to a month's time!

Neuromuscular Reprogramming

Have you ever known someone who got injured, went to rehab, got a clean bill of health, then returned to sport or exercise and reinjured the same area? Yep, I have too. What I find all too often is that when we get injured, the injury was actually brewing for a much longer time before the actual injury occurred. Often if we dig deep enough the person knew something was wrong, was in pain, or just felt “off” and chose to try and train right through it hoping for the best or yielding to the false belief that “maybe it will just go away.” Like I said earlier, your body is a yes man. If we have pain spontaneously disappearing in the body, it’s likely you’re overcompensating on the other side and the injury is persisting even though there is no pain. This rerouting, or reconfiguring of force patterns in the body, needs to be corrected in order for us to permanently heal the injury once we release the fascia without rolling exercises, and then return the muscle to its normal length with our stretching exercises.

For people who have had pain for less than three months, these exercises may not be totally necessary, but will actually compliment your current training regimen because I consider these exercises to be what I call “prehab”—we do them so we don’t get hurt, rather than following the normal course of inaction fighting through pain, getting injured, then having to go to rehab. For those of you who have had pain for 3 to 8 months, you will definitely have to do these exercises, but you will be able to pick and choose which ones serve you best. Lastly, for those of you who have had pain for more than 8 months, you will need to do all of these exercises to make sure you are *reprogramming as many muscles* as possible. Here's why: when we have been in pain for such a long period of time, our tissue not only becomes glued together, and then shortens in length, but it also starts to be used less and less by the body, causing it to atrophy (shrink), and weaken as well. Oftentimes a muscle will not open fully until it gains enough strength to do so. The strength work becomes the missing piece of the puzzle. Once I started instituting strength exercises as part of my protocol for my long time chronic pain clients, their body's ability to heal itself accelerated considerably! This is because all tightness is predicated by weakness.

Weak muscles create dysfunction in our kinetic chain, which promotes movement faults. Release a weak muscle without strengthening it and you will keep on having to release it. Strengthen a muscle while you are trying to release it and it will release and relax, providing permanent relief, and that is what we are truly after. I want you to achieve true motility with your mobility work where you no longer have to think or be afraid of your movement. Another main purpose of my program is to help people develop a permanent mobility practice for the rest of your life! Rather than having to do mobility to get out of pain, you are doing it to prevent pain from arising. I tell people I will spend $500 in prevention to avoid paying 5 or 10 times that in correction.

How much does not being in pain mean to you? Are you willing to mobilize for 5 minutes a day? 20? 45? The answer is different for everyone, but I wouldn't be able to sleep at night if I didn't urge all of you reading this to at least take some care of your body by rolling, strengthening, and stretching at least once per day. I'm not going to say more is better because it is not. Doing 3 hours of mobility is just silly and your body will stop responding past a certain point anyway. I find a solid 20-30 minutes per day is sufficient for most people depending on how much you sit. Ideally we want to do 4 minutes of mobility work for every hour we spend seated. An 8-hour work day, plus sitting in traffic yields about 32 minutes of corrective exercise we need to plan for and make a priority. I've said it before, your body does a lot for you, what do you do for your body?

To perform some of these exercises you will need to buy some special equipment that will set you back a whopping $25 at most. All of the mobility equipment mentioned in this book is available to purchase through Amazon on my website www.influentialhealthsolutions.com/mobility-tools/. Through years of mobility practice I have narrowed down the best tools which will last you the longest. Go cheap on these mobility tools and you will have to keep buying them, spending more money in the long run. Without further adieu let's bring on the strength exercises!

Strengthening The Back

Strength takes on many different meanings in the body. When you think about strength you may picture a man towing a vehicle 50 yards, or a female gymnast holding an iron cross on the rings for a minute. When it comes to the back, strength is displayed primarily as endurance. People rarely lack the strength to move, what they have run out of is the ability to express strength on a long enough continuum. I first saw this at The University of Hawai'i when working with the football team. Our starting running back was complaining of back tightness when running anything longer than a 50-yard spring. This player could deadlift close to 500 pounds—surely he wasn't lacking strength. Doing a simple localized low back muscular endurance test left him cramped up wiggling on the ground for about 5 minutes unable to move. He said it was the hardest thing he has ever done athletically up until that point.

I'm preaching to the choir when I tell you we use our back muscles for everything all day long. Only people who have back pain are unlucky enough to experience this. You'll feel your back muscles activate when you laugh, when you cry, when you sneeze and cough. They will burn when you sit, stand, and lie down. Even the slightest of movements will become a chore to avoid that sting, pinch or dull ache. This makes the primary action of your low back muscles to provide endurance for continuous movement. When our glute, and lower back muscles become tight, not only are we asking them to work harder due to the chronic contraction, but because the capillaries are restricted less nutrients are allowed to come in to help the muscles recover, and less metabolic waste is allowed to be removed from muscle energy production. This produces an unfavorable environment for the back muscles to do their job. Breaking the fascia up, and returning it to its normal length is jobs one and two. After that we then must strengthen it with light resistance repetition after repetition to recondition the muscle. Due to this fact, we will be doing nothing less than

25 repetitions on all of our exercises. As a result, some of you may experience extreme stiffness at first. Your back may burn, and it may be difficult for you to stand up straight. Not to worry, like my friend on the UH football team, your body will eventually clear everything out and you'll be fine. Some people worry about soreness after doing so many repetitions, and for some this may be the case. For the most part, when you get used to doing the exercises the soreness goes away and my clients tell me they wake up with their back feeling looser and more mobile, so do not be afraid to be aggressive. Each individual will progress at their own pace; the most important thing is to finish all of the repetitions as prescribed for said exercise.

Band Walks

Time and time again I have given people this tiny band and asked them to perform the exercise I'm going to describe to you and they can't believe what they feel. Their hips, and low back are burning to the max and they are only a quarter of the way done! It is very simple, yet very effective at the same time.

Muscles Targeted: This exercise works 3 of our primary abductors; the Glute Minimus, Glute Medius, and Quadrattus Lumborum. These are all pelvic stabilizers that support the movement of the low back. When we condition these muscles the lower back will require less involvement and ultimately be a happier camper. If you are a runner, you should do this exercise every day before you run.

How to perform: Lay the band on the floor so there is no tension on it and then step on the band with your feet hip width apart.

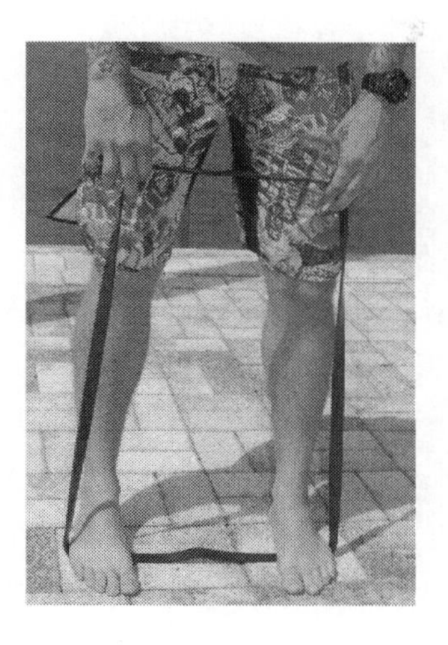

Next, pull the band up and place it around your shoulders, not your neck.

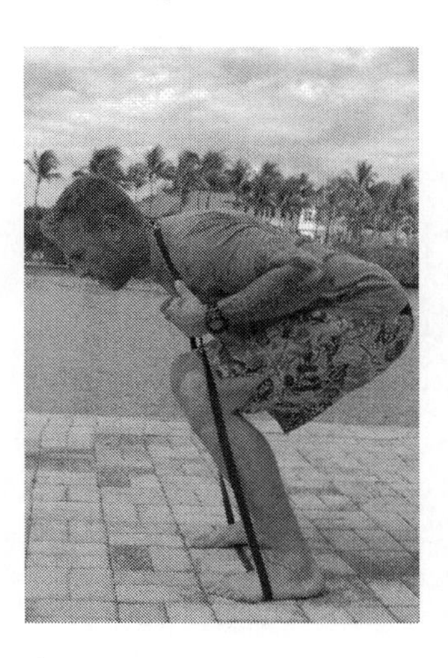

Now space your feet a little further than hip width, spreading the band apart, and making it more tense.

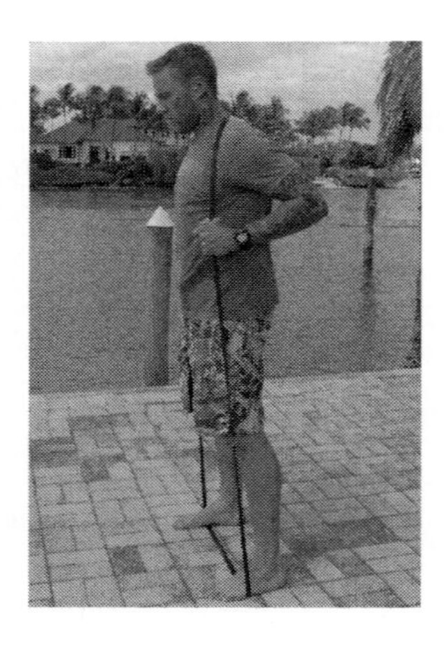

Here comes the challenging part. We now must walk a little more straight-legged than normal to keep the band steady on our feet. Do this for 20-30 feet minimum.

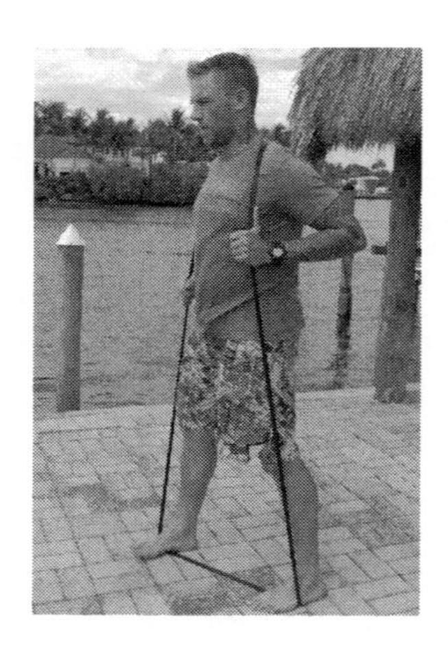

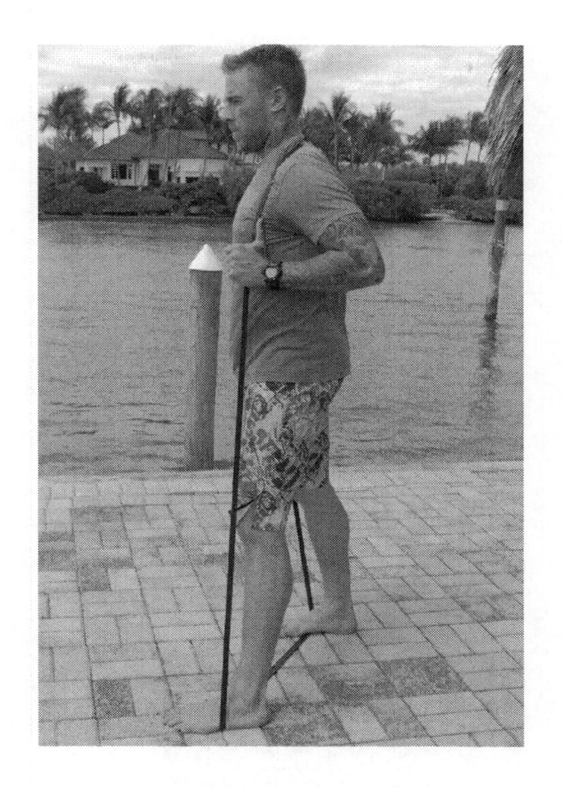

When you reach your prescribed distance, turn to your right. From here extend your right foot away from your body first, and then bring the left foot closer the same distance. Do not bring your feet together. Keep space between them always or else you will make the exercise infinitely more difficult! Return to the starting position stepping with your right foot first, and then closing the gap with the left foot.

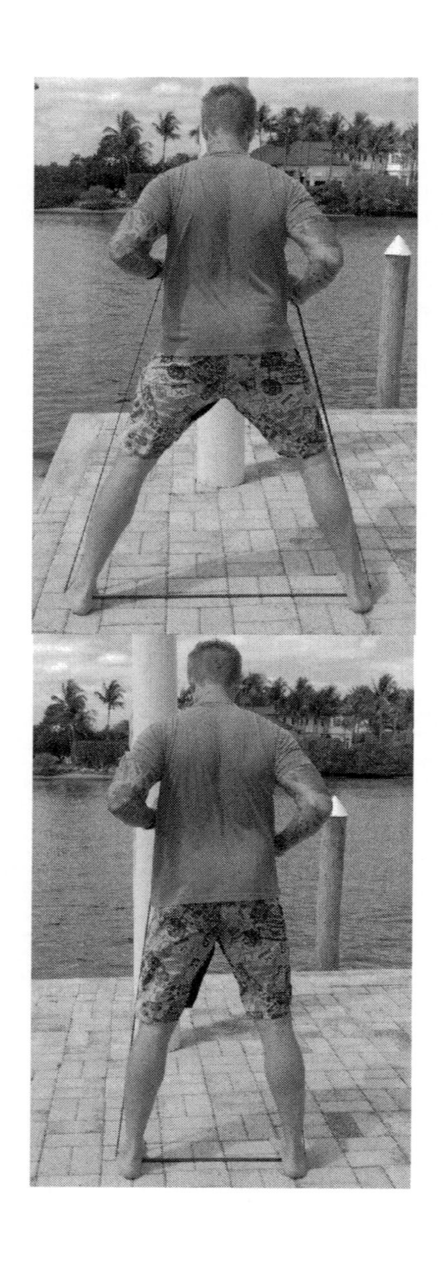

When you reach the starting position, turn downhill and walk with your feet spaced apart again till you reach your prescribed length. This time turn to your left and now we move the left foot away first, then close the gap bringing the right foot closer. Do this all the way back to the start.

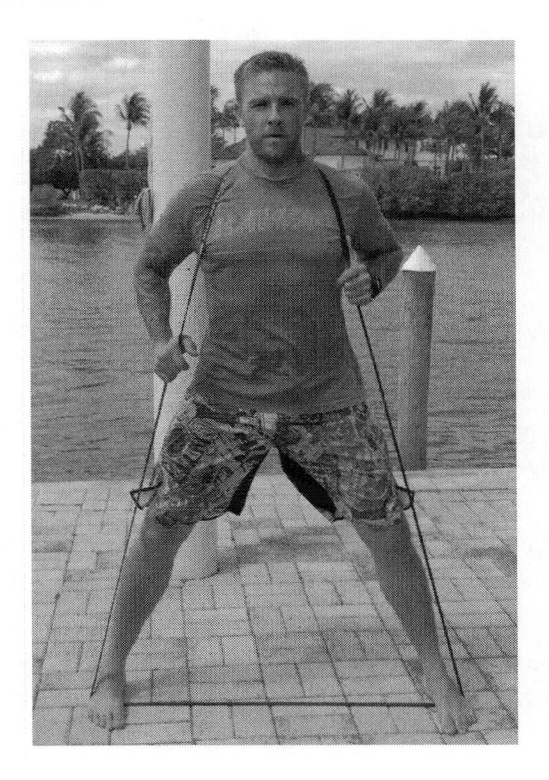

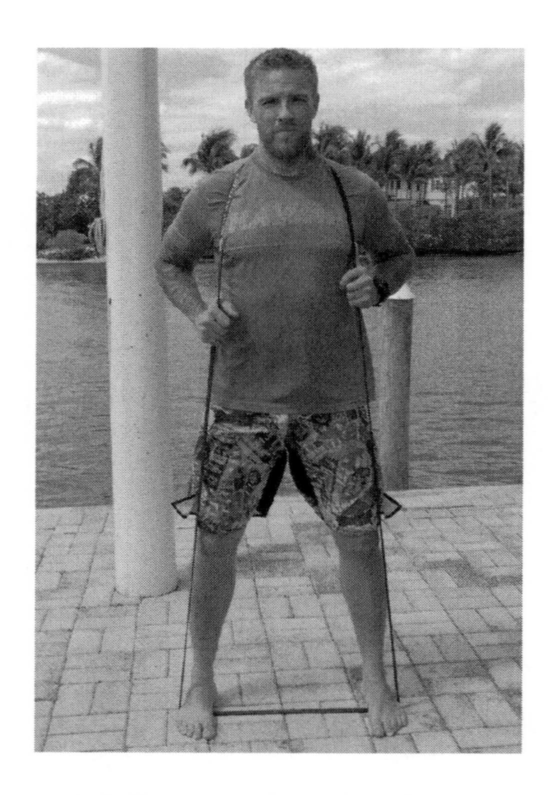

Congratulations, you have just done one repetition. Repeat this 3 times. How long could you do this exercise before your hip and lower back started burning? Take note of where you had to stop and how many times. For some, this exercise may have taken a minute to complete, and for others it could take up to 5 minutes! Fret not, small improvements is all we are looking for on a day-to-day basis. Kaizen!

Deep Hip Hinge Abduction

So simple, yet so challenging to teach, I believe the hip hinge should be mastered in every kindergarten class in the world. Poor form when picking objects up, or sitting occurs from bending at the spine rather than at the hips. The hip hinge teaches you to lock your spine neutral allowing for the greatest expression of strength and endurance.

Muscles targeted: For this exercise are the erector spinae, gluteus minimus, gluteus medius, gluteus maximus, and hamstrings.

How to perform: Place your loop band around your thighs, just above the knees. Keeping your feet directly under your hips, bend the knees slightly, push your butt back and bend over at the hips keeping a rigid spine.

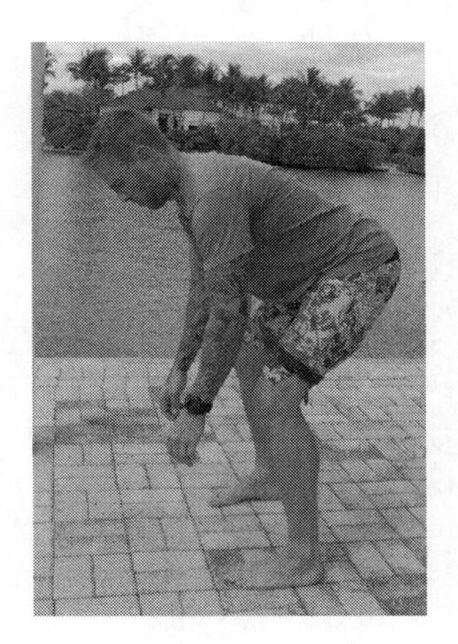

When your torso is parallel to the ground you may now begin the abduction of your legs. Do this by spreading your knees as far apart as possible, and then slowly returning them back to the start position.

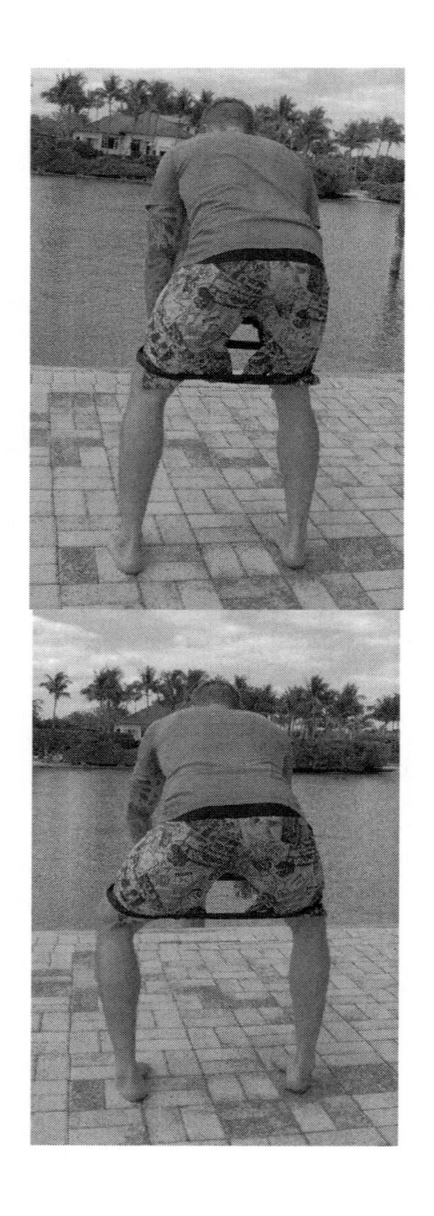

It is important to note we want our knees to go from hip width to outside of our hips, then back to hip width. We do not want to have our knees collapse inward!

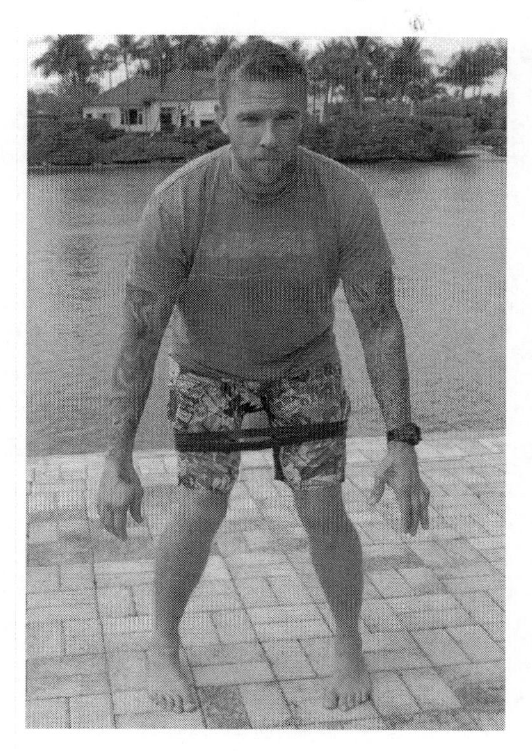

Sets/Reps: Perform 3 sets of 50 repetitions.

I can't emphasize enough how important it is to nail this hip hinge and practice it in your daily movement, not just in your exercise/rehabilitation program. An easy tool to see if you are doing it correctly is to use a PVC pipe or broomstick for feedback. As you hinge, we want three points of contact with the bar on our head, back, and butt. If any one of these points is missing, we are doing the exercise incorrectly, adding stress to our spine. Return to the start position and try again. Go slowly and teach yourself correctly!

Banded Good Morning

Another simple, yet effective exercise to provide localized muscular conditioning to the lower back and supporting muscles is the banded good morning.

Muscles Targeted: We will be training several muscles with this exercise, but where the exercise will be "felt" will depend on how much you are contracting your glutes, and how straight your legs are while performing it. Having said that, the muscles we are targeting with this exercise are the erector spinae, gluteus maximus, and the hamstrings – all hip extensors.

How to perform: Set yourself up with the band as you did in the band walking exercise. Keeping the band relaxed, step on it with your feet hip width apart and then bend down and stretch the band over your head and place it on your shoulders, not your neck.

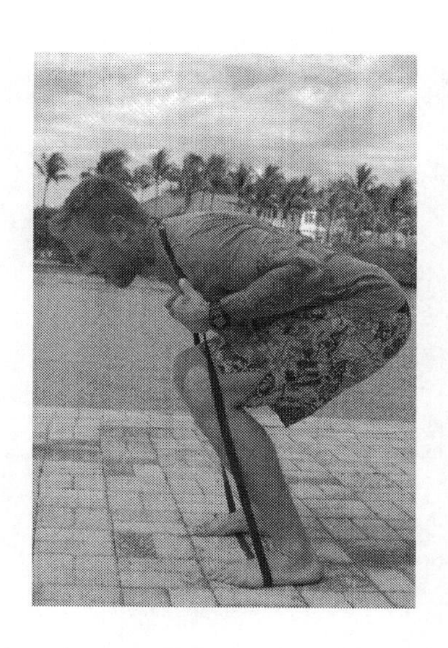

From here we squeeze our glutes first and then release them as we bend over with our knees slightly bent till our torso is parallel with the ground, hinging at the hip as in the previous exercise.

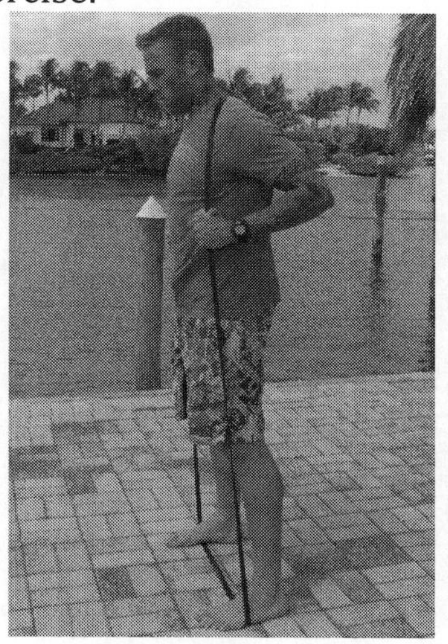

To hip hinge we want to lead with the chest as we descend, not the head. This stops us from curling the back into c-spine which is a huge mechanical no-no.

Back Flat = Good

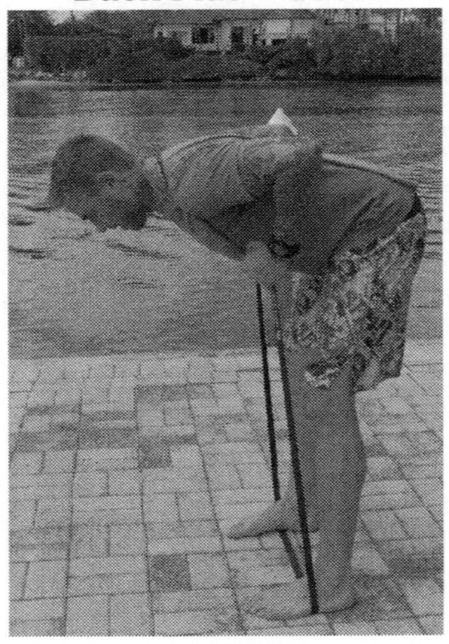

C Spine = No-No

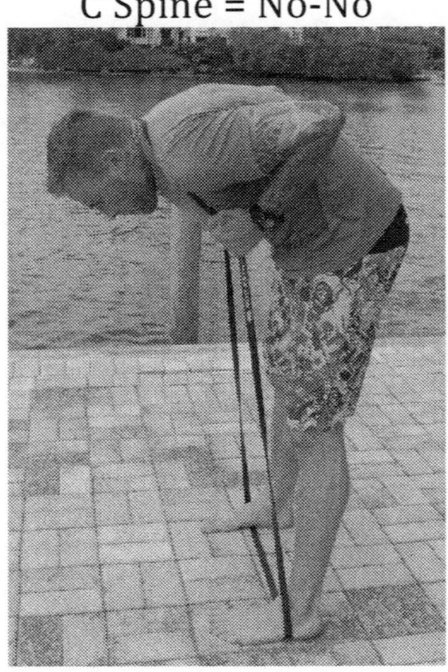

We also want to keep the head in a neutral position. To do this make sure you are looking down slightly as you are descending. Do not bend the neck and look straight ahead on the way down.

Another No-No

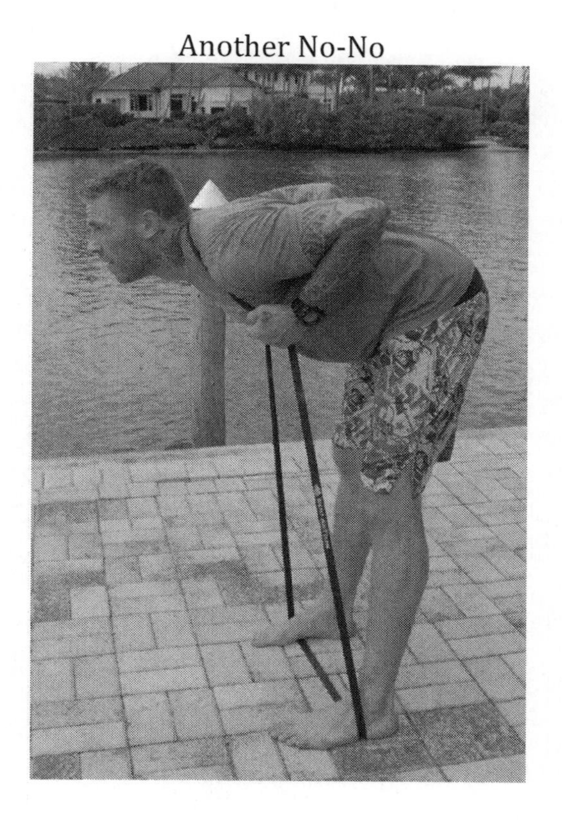

As we return up to the standing position, we want to focus on engaging the glutes first, not pulling from the back. This takes some getting used to, but cueing yourself to think "glutes first," will make a huge difference in how your muscles reprogram. Remember, proper function in the body calls upon the glutes to move first, then the hamstrings, then the lower back last.

Sets/Reps: Perform 5 sets of 30 repetitions, squeezing your butt at the top each time.

Walking Lunges

Believe it or not, walking lunges can be done incorrectly. The main reason for doing a walking lunge is to recruit our gluteus medius to a greater extent and if we do this exercise in an incorrect manner we will not achieve this. In the end we may gain a little more glute and leg strength, but it will not be the right type of glute strength. The gluteus medius, if you remember, is one of the only butt muscles that will refer pain into the back due to trigger points. Strengthening the gluteus medius will make releasing it easier, which makes the importance of doing this exercise greater, and our program more optimal overall.

Muscles targeted: Gluteus medius, gluteus maximus, gluteus minimus, adductors, quadriceps, and the hamstrings.

How to perform:

Start in a standing position with your hands on your hips.

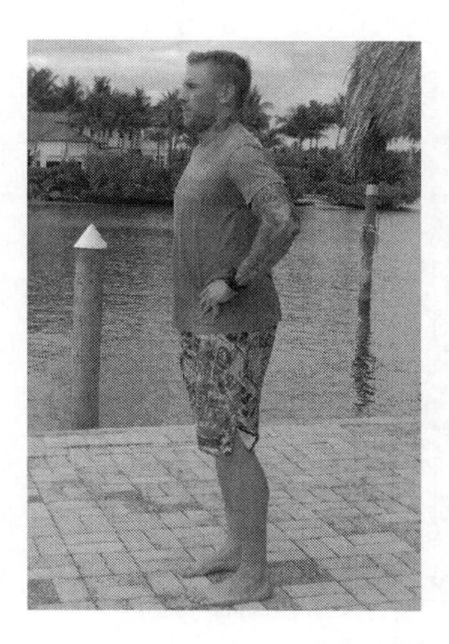

Take a moderately long step and lightly touch your knee to the ground.

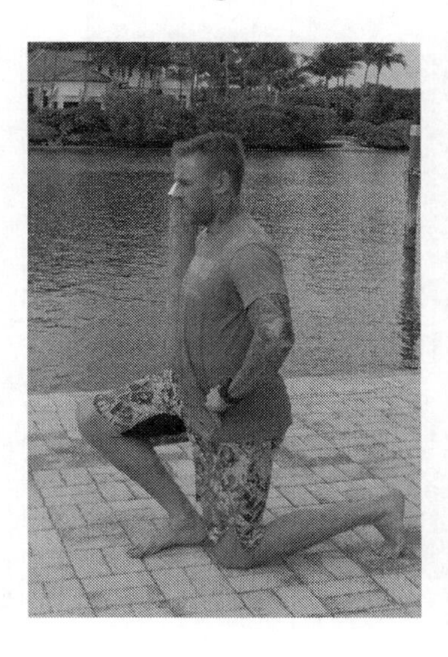

From here take another large step forward without your back foot touching the ground until you are in the lunge position again.

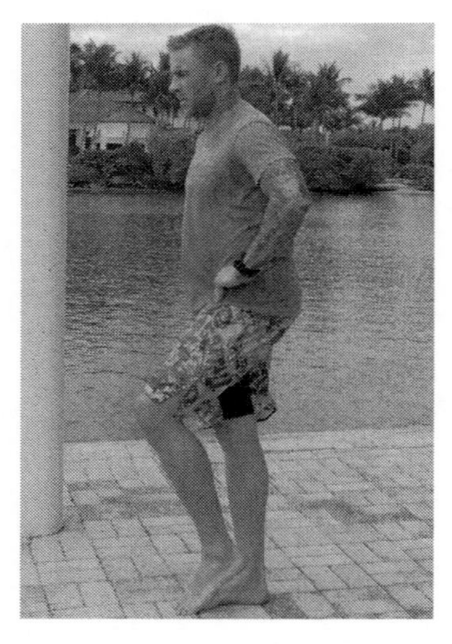

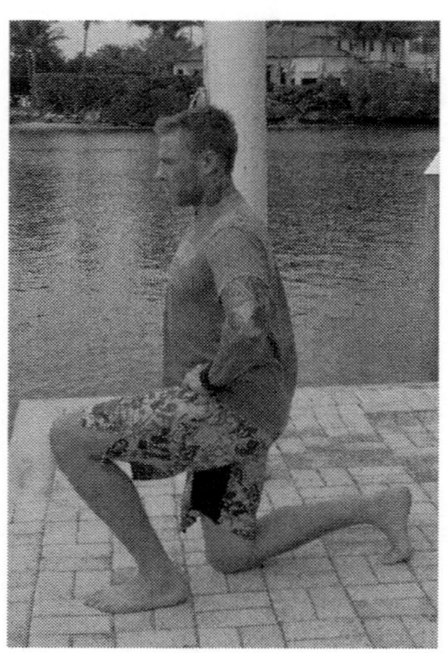

Swinging the leg through fully is what calls upon the gluteus medius for more strength to balance and stabilize the pelvis. Where people go wrong is taking what I call a "false step." Walking lunges should be done like you normally walk. When you walk it is one foot after another. You don't walk, and then place your foot next to the other one. This is the false step I am speaking about.

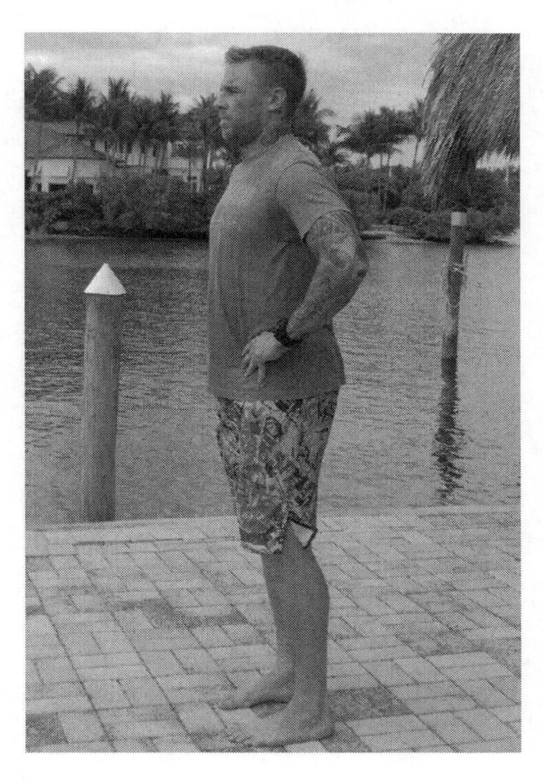

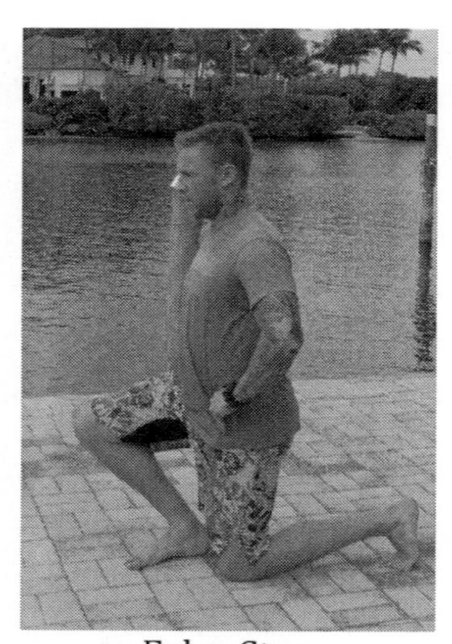

False Step

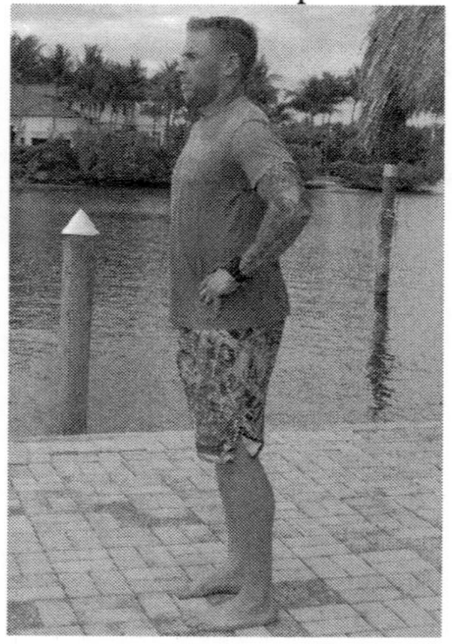

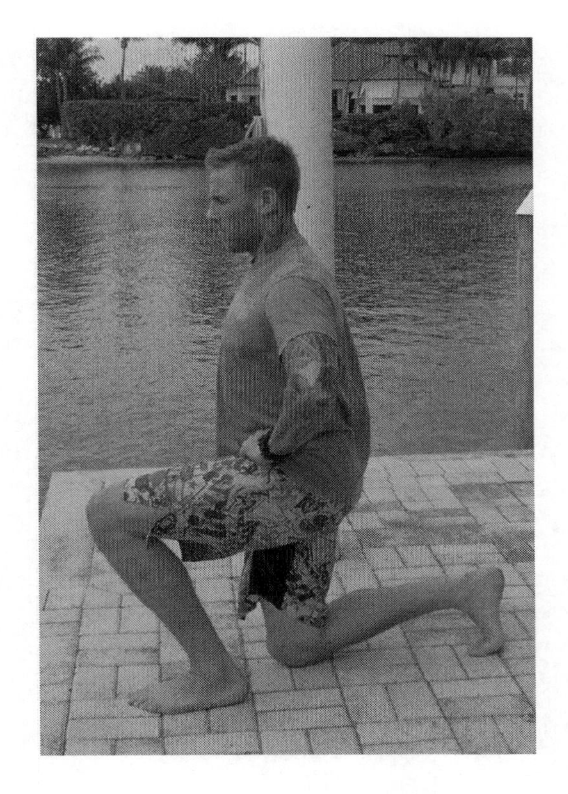

One of the more challenging aspects of this exercise is balance, especially if your gluteus medius is tight and deconditioned. You may be wobbling a bit when lunging but that is okay, just take it slow and make sure you are balanced on the way down. As your glutes get stronger and more conditioned, you will start to balance much easier. I urge you to start off slowly, and focus on sweeping that leg through, rather than taking that false step. Remember, we are reprogramming the muscles. We are actually trying to help them remember what they already know. Like Ida Rolf said, structure is behavior, and proper form will allow proper function!

Sets/Reps: Build up to 5 sets of 10 steps with each leg. Build slowly. If you have never done this exercise before your gluteals will be very sore the next day!

The Four Way Glute Bridge

Your gluteus maximus muscle (the thick fleshy part of your butt) is what physiologists call a quadrilateral muscle, meaning with how the fibers align themselves there are four different angles to it all rolled up into one large muscle. It orients itself from the pelvis to the leg obliquely downward and lateralward. Here is a better picture of what I'm talking about:

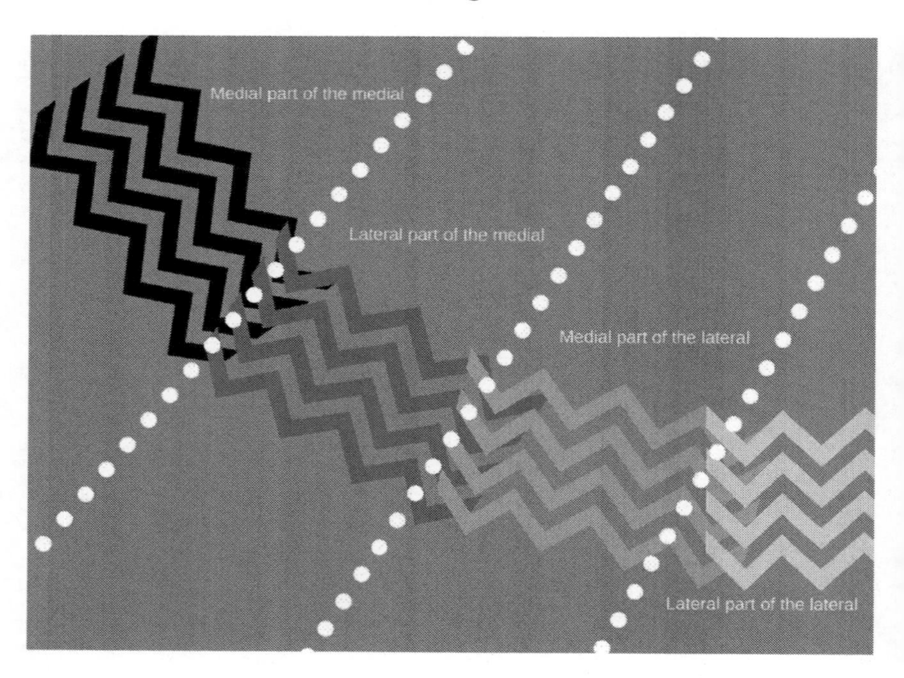

So even though the glute max is one muscle, the fibers go in four different directions. This makes it extremely versatile, yet tricky to train properly if you are not attacking the individual fibers separately. To begin this exercise, we are going to hit the lateral portion of the muscle and then slowly work our way inside to the medial portion.

Muscles targeted: 4 segments of the gluteus maximus, hamstrings, and low back muscles.

How to perform: We are first going to start out isolating the lateral part of the lateral of the gluteus maximus. To do this, lie on your back with your hands in a T fashion.

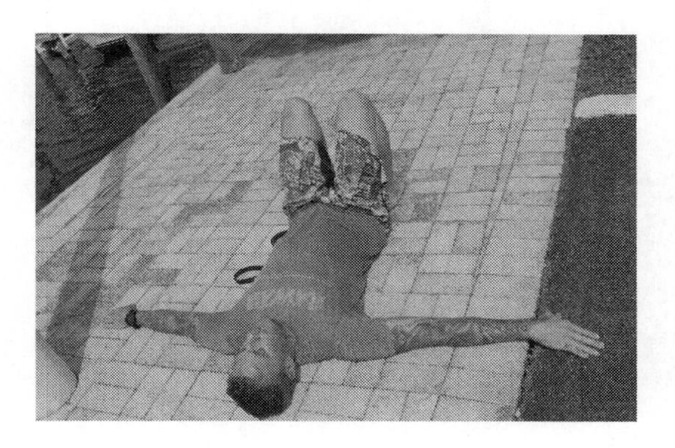

Next, bring your feet as close to your butt as you comfortably can and make sure they are hip width.

Third, place something thin between your knees to squeeze while performing the exercise to make sure you your knee stay together.

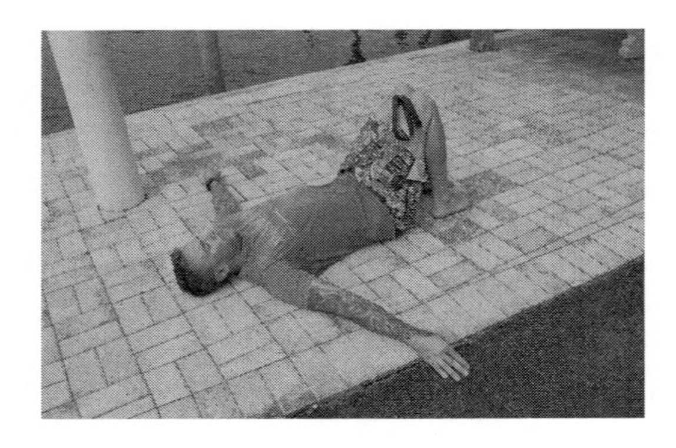

From this position, raise your hips straight up to the ceiling, squeezing you knees together and then finishing off by squeezing your glutes.

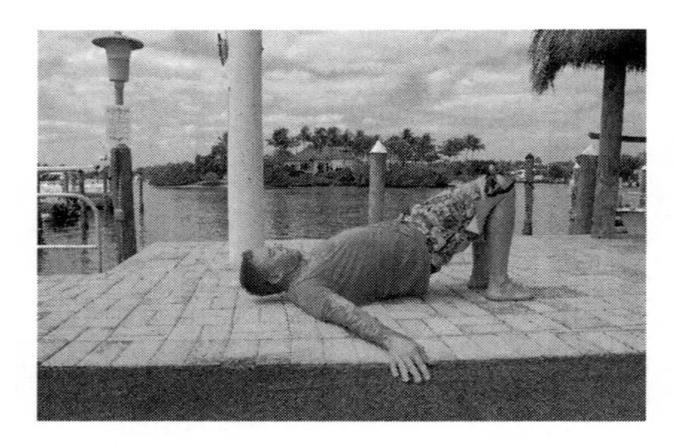

Sets/Reps: Complete one set of 50 repetitions.

We are now going to isolate the medial part of the lateral. To do this we change the position of the feet from being hip width, to touching.

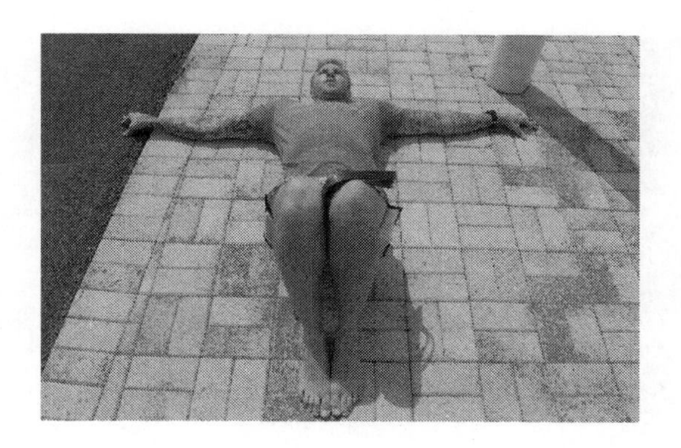

Keep something thin between your knees still to make sure they stay touching. Press your feet into the floor and raise your hips as high as you can, squeezing your glutes at the top.

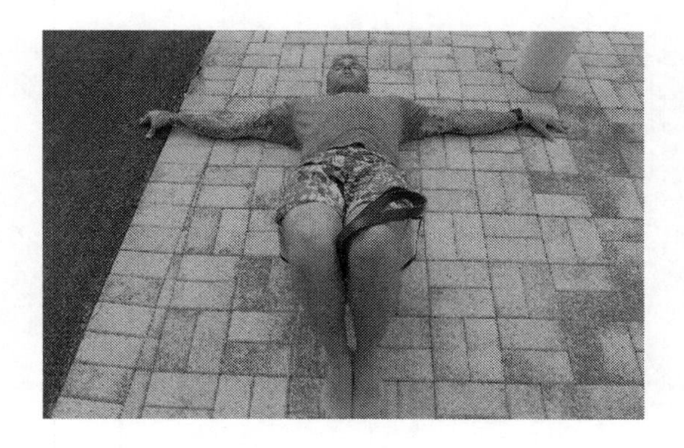

Sets/Reps: Complete one set of 50 repetitions.

Now we are going to work the lateral part of the medial. To do this we want to move the feet back out so they are hip width apart, and then move the knees out so they are hip width apart.

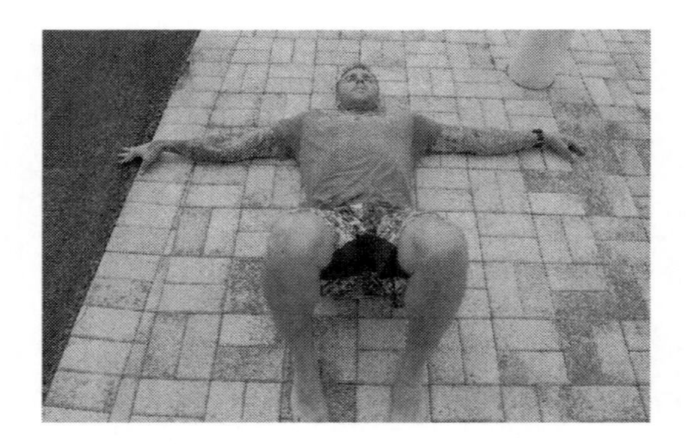

Press your feet into the floor and squeeze your glutes as hard as you can on every repetition, raising your hips as high as you can.

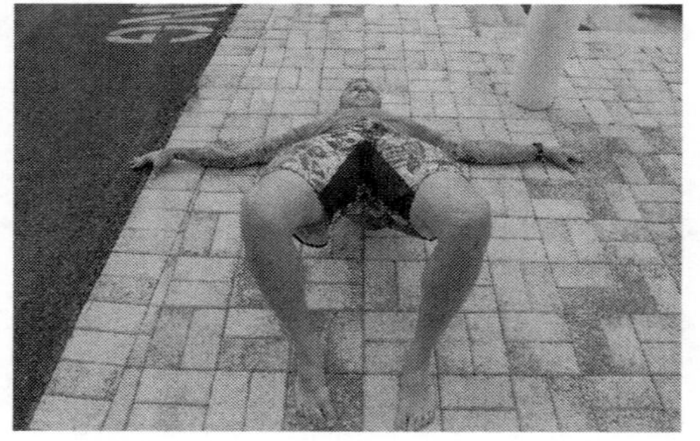

Sets/Reps: Complete one set of 50 repetitions.

Lastly, to hit the medial part of the medial, you are going to move your feet together and then spread your knees apart as far as possible until your feet start coming off of the ground.

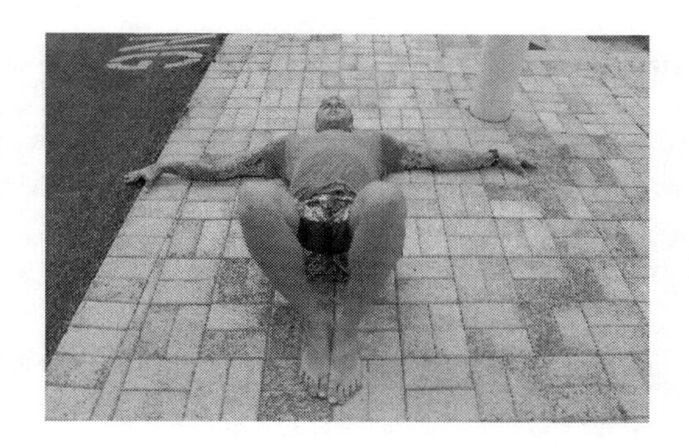

Press your feet into the floor and raise your hips as high as you can, squeezing your glutes at the top.

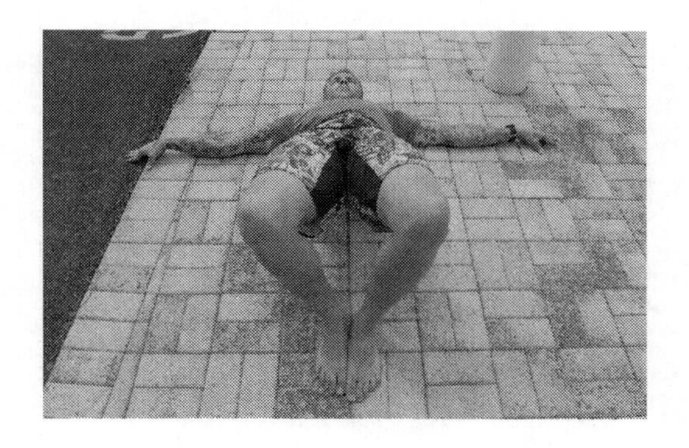

Sets/Reps: Complete one set of 50 repetitions.

And there you have it. This gigantic 200-repetition set should have your glutes burning like an inferno and will probably be the first time some of these fibers were stimulated directly. Word to the wise, I have had athletes and laypeople alike have their hamstrings cramp up on them while doing these exercises. Fear not if and when this happens. Just relax till the cramp goes away, or stand up, walk around, and shake your leg out. In some cases, the stimulation this exercise provides is just a tad bit more than the body is used to handling, but this is the point of exercising – to overcompensate so we don't get injured!

Bent Knee Single Leg Glute Bridge

So far we have been doing a lot of two-legged exercises to strength the back and butt, which is not a bad thing. Doing even one of the previous exercises for the prescribed length, or repetitions is probably more glute work than most of you are used to, but to really reeducate and restore the proper function of the low back we want to separate the body to see if there is a weakness in there somewhere and for the most part the walking lunges we did just won't cut it even though the effect from the soreness may be telling us otherwise.

The bent knee single leg glute bridge is just the right type of exercise to do this for us because it reeducates proper firing patterns all throughout our posterior chain. There are two levels to this exercise, start with level one, and as you progress and the exercise becomes easier, move to level two for an entirely different challenge!
Muscles targeted: gluteus maximus, hamstring, and lower back musculature.
How to perform: To begin level one of this exercise, lay flat on your back with your foot as close to your butt as you can comfortably get it, arms at your sides, and opposite knee in your chest.

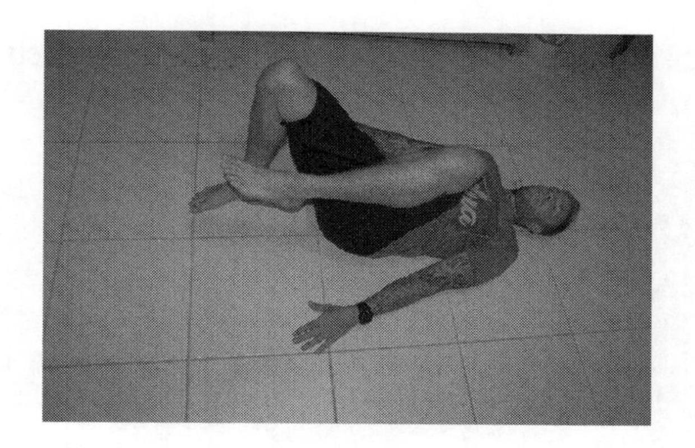

From here, press your foot into the floor and lift your hips to the ceiling as high as possible.

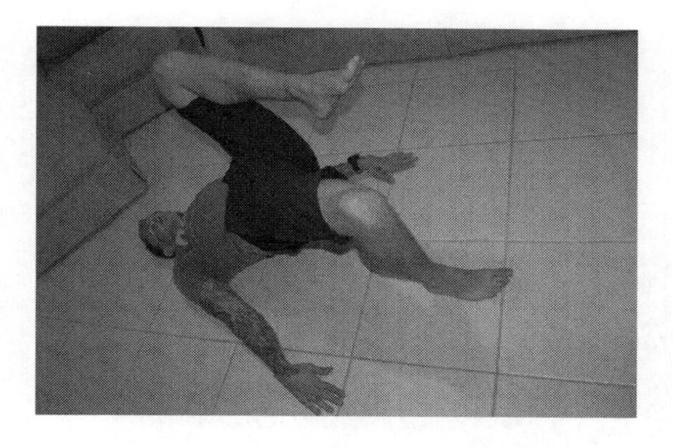

Perform the prescribed number of repetitions on one leg, and then switch to the other leg.

Sets/Reps: 3 sets of 25 repetitions each side.

Level two of this exercise allows us to get into a greater range of motion. To start the exercise, lay on your back with one foot up on a bench or sofa, making sure it forms a 90-degree angle. Draw the opposite knee to your chest and grab your shin keeping your leg close.

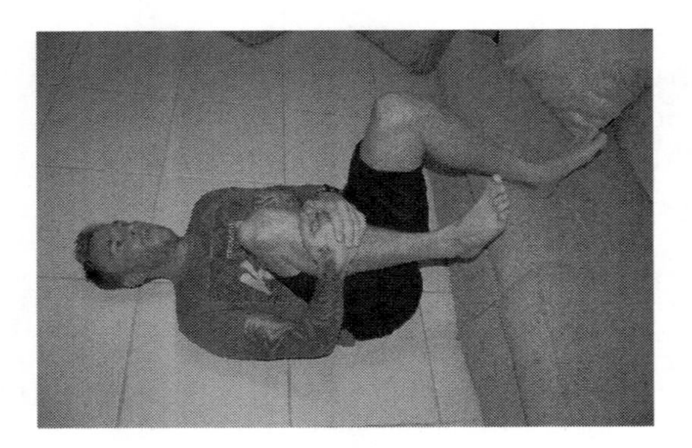

From this position you are going to press your heel into the bench and raise your hips up to the ceiling, locking them out and squeezing your glute as hard as possible, holding the finished pose for a second before you return back to the starting position.

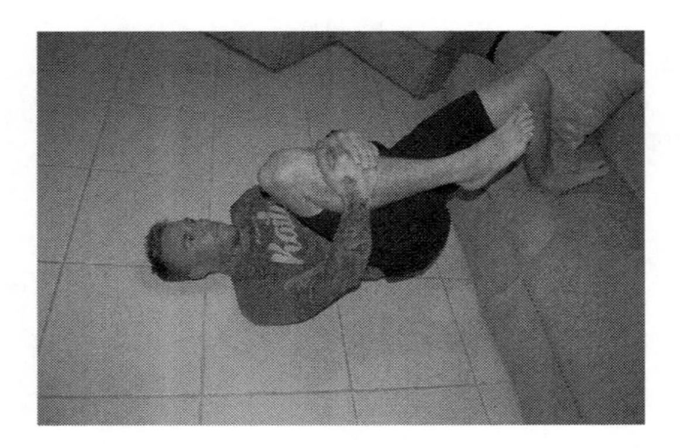

Do all of the prescribed reps on one side before switching to the other.

Sets/Reps: Start off with 3 sets of 15 repetitions. Once that becomes easy, increase to 3 sets of 25 repetitions.

Concluding Thoughts on Strength

Hopefully as you were looking at the pictures and reading the descriptions of the exercises you started to understand where you have gone wrong, and why you ended up on back pain boulevard. For most people, even doing just one set of any of these exercises is enough to cause a negative reaction. Most people will actually feel worse from an exercise that is designed to heal. Why does this happen? We'll cover that a bit more in our "Ask the Coach" section. For now, I want to reiterate our model of healing chronic pain in the body I introduced in the previous chapter. Some of these exercises may provide an extreme benefit to you right away, some of them may be eye-opening and extremely uncomfortable, and there may be one or two your body just isn't ready for yet. Whatever the case is, remember that Rome wasn't built in a day, and we didn't hatch the idea to travel to the moon and accomplish that feat within the first year even. These exercises are designed to get you from a place of pain to a place of power and posture and everyone is starting off at a different point. We must be mindful that people heal differently too. Do not get frustrated. Keep your thoughts positive. Breathe.

Ask the Coach: Why does all of this stuff (rolling, stretching, strengthening) have to hurt? Is that good?

While "no pain, no gain" has been a term that has been the cause of a great many eventual injury, pain does have its capacity to heal; the problem is that pain is largely misunderstood. Thomas Myers, renowned for his work with the human myofascial system and forward thinker of massage therapy has the following definition for pain:

"Pain is sensation accompanied by the motor intention to withdraw."

So if you're not trying to run from it, then technically it is not pain, it is just sensation. To me, pain is not felt only as bad. There is a tremendous amount of good pain I feel through the training, and bodywork I do for myself. While most people share this sentiment, there are a few, not many, but a few that view all pain as bad and have an instinctive desire to avoid it at all costs. To these people I offer the following explanation.

There are three types of pain that we can experience. The first is pain entering the body. This can happen as we fall on a knee ice-skating or bang our thumb with a hammer when we miss the nail. It is usually experienced as physical pain but can be emotional too in the form of witnessing something sad, or horrific. The second type of pain is pain that is stored in the body. This type of pain is often not felt as pain. It's called stress, fatigue, or a feeling of not being able to do something that you wish, want, or used to be able to do. The third type of pain is pain leaving the body. This is the pain we experience through rolling, stretching, strengthening, bodywork, yoga, or weird little exercises that reprogram our butt and make it burn really bad.

Pain leaving the body does so through sensation, but can more aptly be characterized as energy. This energy provides an experience in the experiencer that creates awareness. It is a teacher of sorts on what not to do to be in this position again. It is a reminder when we feel that familiar pain to reach for the foam roller or lacrosse ball as soon as possible because delaying only means more time, and more pain to be lost and experienced in the future. Every one of us has experienced physical pain in some form in our life. Every one of us is walking around with some form of pain stored somewhere in the body as well. Not too many of us are working on releasing this pain, rather we hold onto all of our trauma and drama, absorbing it like a sponge, unleashing it on those we love and hold dear because they are who we are in the closest and most contact with.

Manual therapy (mobility) can now be seen as an alternative way to release emotions, decrease pain, and almost make ourselves cry without actually crying. Stretching can rearrange organs and restore their natural order, helping us digest food better to make the most of our nutrition, bringing proper health and wellness to the entire system. Strength training (muscle reprogramming) can give us a newer, more profound sense of confidence. We may walk with a stronger stride, or not think twice about a random act of kindness (such as opening a door or carrying groceries), which can contribute to the greater collective good of humanity. Seen this way, bodywork seems as though it should be a response-ability for all mankind young and old, for those in pain, and those not in pain. It should be something sought after and revered, rather than something most turn a smug nose to.

The problem is bodywork is challenging and takes time away from our tweeting, trolling of Facebook, or Instagramming. It isn't sexy or cool to be seen rubbing a ball on your inner thigh. It isn't cost-effective to go to a massage therapist and drop $80 to just talk about your relationship and leave covered in oil. To justify the cause we need an effect and I've worked with too many people who were ready to give up before they met me. I hope you are one of those people who see what I have prescribed to already be working. I hope you see its efficacy not blindly, but from the greater ease you are experiencing from your own movement.

Like I said before, I always have a goal and a mission attached to everything I do. My goal is to get you out of pain, and on to a better lifestyle. My mission on the other hand is to change the way your brain thinks about pain and make you realize you are holding the tools to reverse it in your very hands.

Chapter 8 – Troubleshooting

"When health is absent, wisdom cannot reveal itself, and cannot manifest, strength cannot be exerted, wealth is useless, and reason is powerless." –Herophilies, 300 B.C.

Nathan hasn't slept in his bed for the last 5 days. The floor was more comfortable now, and he was getting the feeling that his back pain was serious now. He also has not been to work in the last 5 days either. A single 45-year-old male, if he didn't work there was no other source of income. A friend of his had come to see me a couple months earlier for a shoulder problem and told Nathan that if he wanted to get better fast, I am the guy to go see. Nathan called me and set up an appointment for that afternoon because he needed to get a ride. His back hurt so bad it actually prevented him from being able to drive. As Nathan walked in he was limping slightly, favoring his left leg. He was tall and lanky, and it turns out he was a collegiate rower back in the day. Golf had become a new passion for him and he recently changed jobs as well. He went from teaching physical education at a local high school to dealing blackjack at a casino nearby. He enjoyed the change in pace, and change in pay, but all the sitting he was doing was starting to destroy his back.

As I assessed Nathan, what we found out was that his newfound golf hobby combined with up to 12 hours of sitting dealing cards was creating tightness in his left gluteal his body was just not built to handle. To this date I have never seen a tighter glute amongst any of my clients or athletes. After out first session together Nathan was already able to sleep in his bed. He worked the next day as well, but only for 6 hours. Nathan was 6'6" and weighed 225 pound. The combination of being tall and thin, while rotating and generating a lot of force on his left leg when swinging a golf club created extreme instability for his lower back. As we loosened up his glute and retrained its musculature, his pain became an afterthought in a little less than 4 weeks. He returned to work, golf, and exercise full-time, armed with a generous amount of knowledge about how the body works, and how to fix it when we create dysfunction.

Common Struggles

Did you read and absorb the quote at the beginning of this chapter? If not, go back and re-read it for me. If I were you, I would write it on a sticky note and tape it to the mirror in your bathroom. I tell people pain is a constant reminder of how fragile life is. Hopefully by now you have been trying out some of the movements and putting together a solid mobility practice, if not, you need to get started today! Some of the *common struggles* I see when people start a mobility practice are consistency, patience, and their nutritional lifestyle.

Consistency

No matter how many times I say it, I always get one person here or there who doesn't listen. Here's another great quote to hang on your mirror:
"Just because the pain goes away, doesn't mean you are out of the woods. You are now on the path out of the woods." – Chris Kidawski

If you are doing the mobility exercises and are seeing a reduction in pain, or a stoppage in pain altogether that's great and I'm very happy for you, but this does not mean we stop doing the exercises. I tell people that once the pain goes away, we have probably another month of rolling consistently on our musculature, stretching, and strengthening until we reprogram everything and are finally out of the woods. This means being diligent with our practice everyday. In extreme cases, I may tell someone they need to roll on a muscle 6-8 times a day for at least 2 minutes each time. They look at me with their eyes bugging out in disbelief. The simple fact is when we are not training our muscles to relax; we are training them to re-tighten. Twenty minutes of mobility a day is a small favor your body will appreciate after beating it up for 24 hours.

Another common struggle I see is actually making mobility a daily practice. I get questions like, "How much is too much?" and "Should I do this every day?" My answer is always the same. Your body will tell you how much is enough, and every day you move, you should do mobility. My clients and athletes learn to take mobility as serious as they take their training. The older you are and the harder you train, the harder you have to recover. In your teens, recovery is a some-time thing, in your 20s, recovery should be a part-time thing, and in your 30s and beyond, recovery should be a full-time thing. At 38, my mobility work trumps my exercise 2 to 1. In my mid forties, it may be 3 to 1. All I know is I train every day without pain, and I recover much better when I roll than when I don't. But I've bought in. I've drunk the Kool-Aid. I've recognized the benefit and choose to make mobility a priority in my life. Being consistent means we have to develop new habits. Maybe it's setting your alarm 30 minutes earlier. Maybe it's keeping a roller and a lacrosse ball in your car, or in your office as well as your home. Maybe it's putting it in your calendar every day to help us remember. Hit and miss will not make this program work. Missing one day in 30 is not a very big deal, but doing mobility once every three days, or 3 days on and 2 days off leads down a fast track to nowhere. Movement is never correct 100% of the time, and structure is behavior. Remember these words of wisdom. If we are not working to reverse disease with mobility, then we are inviting it through movement. Something is always better than nothing; just make sure you adhere to the guidelines. A quick mobility session for a tight left glute might look like:

Gluteus minimus smash – 2 minutes
Gluteus medius smash – 2 minutes
Couch Pose stretch – 2 minutes
Single leg Glute Bridge - 1 set of 25 repetitions

That's an astounding 8 minutes you were able to use to retrain your neuromuscular system the proper way to fire! Don't get caught in the trap of, "I'll do it tomorrow." That's taking movement for granted! What if you wake up the next day and the pain has come back, or is way worse than before? We only have the power to control the present; "Tomorrow" is always the fantasyland where a whole bunch of action is supposed to take place. The take home message here is to be consistent. Develop a routine and do not compromise it for anything. If you are in serious pain, getting out of pain is your job away from your job!

Patience

Due to all of the running and jumping I did when I was younger I started to develop considerable patellar knee pain. This is what most of my next book in this series will be about. The condensed version is me realizing I did not have knee pain, I had quad pain. Every trigger point known to man in my quad was active, and sending pain into my knee. As I released the trigger points and cleared out my muscle, the pain in my knee was diminishing greatly, but there were some very resistant knots that would not leave. I remained patient however, and what I found was quite amazing. In some cases, it took up to three months of putting the same amount of pressure, in the same spot, for the same amount of time for the tissue to release. In other cases, it took 6 months. And in yet other cases, it took up to a year of constant reprogramming for the muscle to finally let go! I have no scientific rationality for it, but this is sometimes the case. You can roll in the proper area, with the proper pressure for the proper time, and then one year later the muscle finally decides to relax and let go. It's tough to have this kind of patience because at times you just want to give up and convince yourself you are just wasting your time. Don't you believe it! This is resistance at its finest. Be patient. Relax and breathe through the exercises. Visualize your muscles letting go. Send positive mental energy to every cell of your body. Don't get frustrated. All good things, and all great changes take time to develop. Adhere to our method, modality, and time principles and if the muscles you are working on refuse to give up that day, save your energy and inspiration for the next day, or the day after that. I promise your patience will pay off!

Nutrition

There are not too many people that take the, "You are what you eat" phrase too literally. But when you look at it, we are all exactly what we eat. To slam-dunk my point, we are going to use NBA all-star Derrick Rose as an example. He is a self-proclaimed junk food addict. He boasted having a custom made skittles machine in his home with three years of skittles inside of it and many of his college and professional teammates comment on never seeing Derrick eat an actual meal, only junk food. In April of 2012, Derrick tore his left anterior cruciate ligament and since then has gone on to have two more knee surgeries on his right knee, and as of the writing of this book he is set to have another surgery on his left knee.

So what gives?

When we look at our body, we see one unit as a whole. When we look under our skin, as mentioned in the earlier chapters, we see our body really is one cohesive unit all the way down to our bones. Dissected, we can see our lovely fascia, blood vessels, nerves, muscle tissue, tendon, ligaments, and organs. What we fail to see and recognize is that we still are not made up of those things. On the most basic level we are a collection of trillions of cells that are regenerating on a daily basis (If you really want to get cosmic with this, we are technically a specific arrangement of atoms, which are mostly space. We are told we are mostly water, which from an observational standpoint is true, but on a microscopic level we are mostly made up of.... space). The cells that make up all of the structures of our body are replicated using the energy we get from the food we eat. If you replace parts on your car from a junkyard, will you expect them to perform like a new part fresh from the factory?

Of course not.

This leads us into the question, "Do I want my cells to replicate using refined sugars, chemicals, and bleached oils as building blocks?" Or, "Do I want my cells to replicate using grass fed beef, wild caught fish, a ton of fresh vegetables, and some fruits and nuts?" To some people fuel is fuel when it comes to their body. But nobody would use the same gas in a jet as they would in their lawnmower. That would be silly. We need to eat what nature has made for us, not what some chemists concocted during a quarterly board meeting. The food we eat literally makes the contents of our cells, which is called protoplasm. Protoplasm is the living contents of our cells. This includes the nucleus and all of the organelles. I hope you're getting a picture of just how deep our nutrition affects how our body feels, how resilient the structures will be because of it, and of course how much energy we will have for specific tasks or different levels of exercise. Derrick isn't falling apart because of age, or because he is unlucky, his body is failing him because as a high level athlete (think jet) he is putting fuel in his body fit for a lawnmower. I believe he is getting injured due to malnutrition!

Nutrition is one of the most difficult aspects for some of us to change or control. I have worked with many people over the course of my coaching career looking to lose weight and have a great many success stories. The challenging aspect is mainly peer pressure. The husband wants to lose weight, but the wife does not and continues to fill the house with grains and pastries. The friends you used to go drinking with every Friday, Saturday, and then Sunday afternoon don't call you anymore because weight loss and alcohol are not symbiotic. Your co-workers egg you on, or think you're narcissistic because you won't have a piece of cake for Jane's birthday at 2 in the afternoon. Changing your nutrition takes a great deal of understanding who you are, and how you want to live. For me, $500 in prevention is worth $500,000 in correction. Is that cake worth the lifetime cost of a heart attack at $130,000? Many of us don't think like this though. We live in the moment, or figure we'll just hop right back on the diet tomorrow, but we don't. Dieting can often be just as destructive with the "lose 30 pounds in 30 days" claims where you drink a solution that was sitting in a plastic bottle for who knows how long. I could go on for a very long time about this stuff, as I'm sure you are starting to notice. If you would like to learn more about food and nutrition, how it controls you, how to make better choices to lose weight, end allergies, and restore strength and elasticity to you muscles and connective tissue, you can pick up my book, *The Death of Dieting* on Amazon.

I hope you have considered what I spoke about in this section greatly. Changing your food choices will power your cells in ways you never thought possible. We all have the ability to fly high, the problem is most of us are using fuel fit for a lawnmower!

Stress Levels

Stress these days is much different than the stress our ancestors evolved with. Today stress is everywhere from the TV, to our work schedule, to an impending divorce, to something we see on Facebook. It could be the light in our bedroom, or the noise coming from a neighbor. Sometimes it can be your own family creating a lot of your stress. To combat stress, many of us are encouraged to exercise, which does have its benefits, no doubt. But the fact is that exercise too can be a stressor, and because it is a catabolic activity means that it is breaking down our body's structures, not just building them up. One of the other ways for us to combat stress—one that is gaining popularity these days—is meditation. I mentioned it already in chapter one, and gave some recommendations, but would like to state my case clearer here because I know it can be of benefit for you.

A simple Google search will return a laundry list of benefits that meditation provides for the mind, body, and soul, so it need not be repeated here. One thing we do need to understand is that meditation has been very successful in helping people get rid of—you guessed it—chronic pain. This is because meditation actually increases the amount of stress our body can handle naturally. If your stress levels remain the same, but you have a greater ability to handle it, it will feel as if your stress is actually diminishing. Many people have trapped emotions they have not worked out for many, many years. This trapping of emotions can be deadlier than any cancer, or virus, because it affects every cell from the inside out; especially the way we think. When we change the way we think about pain, and realize it may be coming from somewhere else besides our muscles, we can cure pain instantly in some cases. This is what Peter Levine and Maggie Phillips discuss in their book *Freedom from pain: Discover your body's power to overcome physical pain.* Although they don't directly talk about meditation, they do recommend a lot of meditation-like exercises. They talk about clearing bad energy, and bring in good energy. They explain how the chemicals formulated in the brain by a bad thought can manifest themselves in the body within 20 seconds! When we are in pain, we see our body as the enemy. Once again using a mechanical reference, if our car breaks down, we don't think our car hates us. I have listened to my clients tell me all about how they think their body actually hates them. They are their body! Neurons that fire together wire together and the more they fire, the more we strengthen the signal. Thinking that our pain is "killing" us provides a lot of negative feedback strengthening the pain signal.

Meditation will work in several ways, but none more so than our breath. Stress constricts our ability to breathe and open our lungs fully, which keeps us in a heightened, contracted state. For some people, one of the simplest things they can do before going to bed to help them sleep is blow up a balloon. Sounds silly right? What this does is get us out of that stressed out position where we are always inhaling or gasping in short breaths. Blowing up a balloon shifts our body from a tense inhalation, to a relaxing exhalation. There are many guided meditations you can find on the Internet, especially YouTube, and this is where I recommend you begin. Most people who have not meditated before lose interest if there is nothing to follow. Guided meditations are like having your own personal coach, and it also gives you a fixed amount of time to meditate. This can be for as little as 5 minutes, to as long as 30. Pick which best suits you. Often times the hardest thing for us to do is get out of our own way. Some of us fear losing control over what we perceive, or have come to know as true. Who will we be without this pain? What will people expect from us now? These are all things meditation helps us with. Meditation increases our awareness we have in our life, which increase the amount of choices we see available. Nobody consciously chooses to be in pain, but when we think all hope is lost and give up, we start to recognize the pain as being a part of us, which it is not.

One of the easiest meditations we can do for 5-10 minutes after waking up is called a Vagus nerve meditation. Our Vagus (Vagus means "wanderer") nerve is the longest nerve in our body, is connected to the most organs, and also stimulates our vocal chords as well. Our Vagus nerve is very closely tied to our emotions, especially traumatic events by stimulating norepinephrine production in the amygdala, the survival part of our brain. When we have chronic pain, we may have a decreased vagal tone, which is not allowing our body to return to a normal, relaxed state thus allowing pain to persist. When vagal tone is high we have less stress, a better mood, decreased pain, and better digestion. To increase your vagal tone you can do what is called a "loving kindness" meditation. There are several of them on the Internet, but here is what I do. The first five minutes of my meditation I do everyday includes feeling a deep sense of gratitude for my entire Vagus nerve. Start at the base of your skull and then pretend to trace your Vagus nerve all the way down your body. Have gratitude for your speech, your heart, your lungs, your diaphragm, your pancreas, your kidneys and all of your digestive organs. This sense of gratitude or thanks that you perpetuate into your own body is like getting a thank you card from your boss for a job well done. It's great to give thanks to God or the Universe for all of the blessings in your life, but what about your own body? Your mind will achieve what you believe, remember.

If you wake up shunning your pain and being depressed over it, your brain will reinforce the pain believing that is what you want, but if you wake up everyday giving thanks that your body is doing its best for you, a much different signal is being sent. A 2010 study by Barbara Fredrickson and Bethany Kik found that increasing positive emotions led to increased social closeness, and an improvement in vagal tone. Not only will you deal more pleasantly with yourself and your body's shortcomings, but you will be able to deal with others much more easily as well.

To me it all makes sense. Treat yourself poorly, and you get poor results. Treat your body with kindness and positivity and you will get positive results. Is meditation a silver bullet? No. But it will help you not only with your pain, but also with a lot of other things in your daily life. Meditating for a minimum of 10 minutes a day can change the way you think and feel tremendously. I call it taking out your mental garbage because it allows you clear all of the worry, and negative feelings out before your day begins. Others call it Zen. Some call it clearing your mind. Whatever label you give it, meditation has been proven effective for thousands of years now; maybe you should start giving it a try!

Supplements

I'm not a massive fan of supplements because people feel they can be a replacement for actual food, exercise, or proper rehabilitation. The way I see it, if there's a pill, there's still a problem. Having said that, there are some supplements that are necessary because no matter how well you try to balance out your diet, or no matter how much sun you try to get, our food, and your position from the equator just will not allow you to get enough. Thus, some supplements become necessary, but with all of these supplements companies out there selling us snake oil, who can you trust not to make your money disappear, rather than your pain? Below is a short list of trusted supplements I use and what I use them for. For a more complete list you can go to https://influentialhealthsolutions.com/chris-approved-products/.

Product – **Ease Magnesium by Activation Products**

What's it for – Pain management, and sleep

How to use it – Spray 10-15 sprays on any area affected with pain, stiffness, or common cracking and popping. The reason I love this product is because of the ease of its use. Spray on 5 minutes before climbing into bed and forget about it. Magnesium oil works better than pills because you are not losing any through the process of digestion. Taking too much oral magnesium will also cause disaster pants (a.k.a. diarrhea), but this will not happen with magnesium oil because the skin will regulate the uptake. When your body has enough magnesium it will simply stop absorbing it. This product is a necessity because sadly, there is no longer enough magnesium contained in the food we eat. Nearly everyone is deficient in this mineral and these deficiencies can be pretty epic in our body because magnesium is responsible for energy production, protein formation, gene production, and it calms the central nervous system. That's a lot of important stuff I just don't want to mess with. Ease Magnesium is a mainstay in my program, and it should be in yours too.

Product – **Vitabreeze Pure Turmeric Curcumin**

What's it for – Pain management, reduces inflammation, anti-carcinogenic.

How to use it – While the verdict is still out on curcumin scientifically, I have had tremendous results with it when it comes to managing pain, and inflammation in the human body. I have seen post surgical knees get reduced by half their size just a day or two after surgery even without the use of ice! Curcumin come from the root turmeric and is also being looked at as an anti-carcinogenic. Most studies show 1,500 mg per day before bed to be giving the best results. Getting it with Bioperine increases its effectiveness and many manufacturers are already selling a combination of the two.

Product – **Sports Research Vitamin D**

What it's for – Soft tissue health

How to use it – A fat-soluble vitamin, it turns out Vitamin D actually acts like a hormone in the body. It is released by the skin when we are exposed to the sun, but most of us are not exposed nearly enough to reap our body's own manufacturing of it thus supplementation is the only viable option. There has been much debate over the safest amount to be ingested due to the fact that fat-soluble vitamins tend to stick around in the body longer than water-soluble vitamins like Vitamin C. The FDA bumped its recommendation from 1,000 IUs per day to now 5,000. I recommend 15,000 per day. Don't be worried about toxicity, some studies have shown no ill effects on 25,000 IUs per day for up to 3 years. Studies have also shown that a majority of athletes that have reoccurring soft tissue injuries end up being tested to have low vitamin D levels. This information alone made Vitamin D a mainstay in my supplement cabinet, and it should be in yours as well. Make sure to take it in the morning time, because Vitamin D is contraindicated with melatonin production—our sleep hormone—so taking it at night might cause you to toss and turn and not sleep very well.

Ask the Coach: How Important Is Sleep?

Sleep disorders add $16 billion dollars to national healthcare costs each year, and sleep-deprivation-caused accidents in the workplace add another $134 billion. Is sleep important? HELL YES! But why? Sleep is important for two reasons:

1. The brain clears up cellular garbage when you sleep.
2. The body repairs itself while you sleep.

You see, after a long day of trivial tasks, your brain is full of bits and pieces of information. Some need to be organized and kept; some need to be thrown out. Your brain is the best computer in the world... tomorrow! Not today. If we don't sleep we eventually lose space to store new information. When this happens our body begins to malfunction in the following ways:

- Problems regulating body heat.
- Immune system decline.
- Increase in stress hormones, and if stress becomes chronic your body will decrease the amount of gray matter in the brain that deals with rational thought.
- The hormone Ghrelin runs rampant, stimulating your hunger and we end up getting fat.
- Inflammation skyrockets.

If we are not sleeping enough, we are not helping our body release growth hormone and testosterone to repair the damage we did to our muscles. So next time you try to train on 2 hours of sleep, know you are shrinking your brain, shrinking your muscles, and making yourself sick!

How much sleep do we need?

According to the National Sleep Foundation, adults should get 7-9 hours of sleep, and children between the age of 10-17 should get 8.5-9.5 hours per night! Oddly, for adults, sleeping more than 9 hours is related to increased risk of chronic disease, and a shorter life. Check out these stats on sleep deprivation and performance:

- Max bench dropped 20 pounds after 4 days of restricted sleep.
- With proper sleep tennis players hit the ball 42% more accurately.
- Losing sleep equates to an 11% reduction in time to exhaustion.
- Perceived exertion increases 17-19% after losing a total of 30 hours of sleep (meaning exercise feels harder).

Let's face it: we are a nation that prides itself on its busy-ness. We think 2 hours of sleep and 16 hours of work is going to get us to where we want, but the body has its limits. What we fail to do is make sleep a priority. We know it's a necessity, but so is food. Eat bad food and we get bad energy. Sleep poorly and your performance will drop eventually. When we are in pain we need to make sleep a priority. Sleep is when we recover. Sleep is when you allow the body to heal itself. From this day forward, I urge you to make a conscious decision to not only get more sleep, but better quality sleep as well. You won't regret it!

Chapter 9 - Putting It All Together

"So many people spend their health to gain wealth, and then have to spend their wealth to regain their health." –A.J. Reb Mater

Richard came to me with pain in the right side of his back he has been dealing with for over 25 years. Asking him about his history, he described to me the fateful day with surprising detail. He could remember the weather, where he was, and even what he was wearing. He was picking his newborn up from a chair. As he turned to reach down and pick his baby boy up, he twisted again on the way up and heard a little pop, then a rush of pain to the area. Richard rested for about two weeks as the pain decreased, then went back to his regularly scheduled exercise. He was never the same. One day his back would ache in the area, another day it was pinching, and yet another day it would be stabbing. It was a roller coaster of pain, some days lighter than others, but it was never fully gone. Not one for doctors, he took to seeing a chiropractor in hopes that the adjustments would help whatever was wrong. After two years he realized he wasn't getting any better, and futility started to settle in. This may be something I just have to deal with, he thought.

Our first assessment uncovered an extremely tight left glute, and some pretty serious scarring in the right lower back. Our first order of business was to return that left glute to its normal length. Once that glute was open we could attack the lower back and get that to calm down too. Richard took to rolling and stretching the left glute, as well as rolling out the entire fascial sheet of his back, concentrating on the lower right side to break up the adhesions. Within 6 weeks Richard was pain free. He still does his glute and back strength training exercises every day, realizing it's easier to stay well than it is to get well!

If the Pieces Fit

Nothing works without structure. At least not optimally, and I want my program to be optimal for you. This section is dedicated to being a quick reference guide for you to look at before you start each session.

Rule #1 – Always roll before you stretch; this makes stretching 10x more productive.

Rule #2 – Always roll and stretch before you strengthen. We want to reset the body before we reprogram. Rolling and stretching will place the muscles in a better position, and will help them remember their own neuromuscular firing pattern. This breaks down and corrects the old incorrect firing pattern.

Rule #3 – Always use the proper modality (ball, roller, etc.), and the minimum effective time is 2 minutes; anything less than that and we are wasting our time.

Rule #4 – When stretching, slow going in, slow coming out. Inhale before, exhale during. Stretch actively, not passively.

Sample Program

So how do we fit all this stuff in? Simple. When people are in pain I tell them their only job is to get better, which means all the exercises in this book become your other full-time job besides your job, your family, or any other obligations you have on a day-to-day basis. Remember to be consistent; even 10-20 minutes a day is better than nothing. Here is what a 7-day program may look like.

Monday

- Abdominal mobility – 10 minutes.
- Hip flexor mobility – 6 minutes each side.
- Hip flexor stretch with rotation – 2 minutes per side.
- Walking lunges – 3 sets of 10 repetitions each leg.

Tuesday

- Gluteus minimus mobility – 4 minutes each side.
- Gluteus medius mobility – 4 minutes each side.
- Lower back mobility – 10 minutes.
- Modified lunge stretch – 2 minutes per side.
- One full set of band walks.
- Deep hip hinge abduction – 3 sets of 50 repetitions.

Wednesday

- Gluteus maximus mobility – 6 minutes per side.
- Hamstring mobility – 4 minutes per leg.
- Low back mobility – 10 minutes.

- 75-90-120 Glute stretches – 1 minute at each position per leg.
- Banded good morning – 5 sets of 30 repetitions (squeeze your butt at the top!).

Thursday

- Hip flexor mobility – 4 minutes per side.
- Gluteus medius mobility – 4 minutes per side.
- Hip flexor with rotation – 2 repetitions of one minute per side.
- Couch pose stretch – 2 repetitions of 2 minutes per side.
- Four-way glute bridge – 1 set of 50 repetitions in each plane.

Friday

- Abdominal mobility – 6 minutes.
- Hamstring mobility – 4 minutes per side.
- Low back mobility – 10 minutes.
- 75-90-120 stretch – 2 minutes in each position per side (stretch the tight side twice).
- Bent knee single leg glute bridge – 3 sets of 15 repetitions per leg.

Saturday

- Hip flexor mobility – 4 minutes per side.
- Gluteus minimus mobility – 4 minutes per side.
- Hip flexor with rotation stretch – 3 sets of one minute per side.
- One full set of band walks.

Sunday

- Gluteus maximus mobility – 6 minutes per side.
- Hamstring mobility – 4 minutes per leg.
- Low back mobility – 10 minutes.

- Van Dammes – 3 sets for 1 minute trying to get lower each time.

I know I've been doing this a lot longer than you, but hopefully you can pick up on the pattern I was using. Two or three mobility exercises, one stretching exercise, and one strength exercise. On a side note, whenever I mobilize the hip flexors or abdominals, I always like to stretch them that day as well.

My Wish for You

Everybody is different, but the same. We all have our own story to tell about our pain and the things we have been through in our life. The one thing we all share in this life is that we all experience pain. Some of us recover faster than others from pain, and in some cases we heal in the same amount of time, but take different roads to get there. I sincerely hope the message I put forth in this book helps you see the body from a different perspective. I hope you see how delicate it is, and also how complex. You may start this program with a family member or friend and they may get better before you. Maybe you heard about someone else healing in half the time. Do not be discouraged. Be patient and work diligently at getting better and you will. A Chinese proverb reminds us to never mock progress, no matter how slow. *My wish for you* is that everything in this book comes easy to you. That you feel a major difference from day one. That the knowledge presented breathes new life into you and brings hope for a happy, pain free future.

The pain we all experience is for us to remember and appreciate how good life truly is to us when we treat our bodies, and life, with respect. Disrespect your body and it will rebel no doubt, but as adults these are conscious decisions we are making so we hold all of the guilt and shame. It's very easy to blame your job, your commute, your family, the wrong play your coach called back in high school, or a defect in the mattress you bought. The tough part is ownership. Owning up to the fact that we are in pain because of the way our brain thinks about it. Owning up to the fact that we bought into someone else's idea of pain that doesn't quite serve you and the direction you want to go in your life. We listen to other people's stories and have the ability to feel compassion for them, but where is our compassion for ourselves? We get frustrated and angry and give up. My final message is to help you realize that as long as you're holding this book you are holding the key to live a pain free lifestyle, because your journey with me does not end here; it's just beginning.

Ask the Coach – How Do I Become a Client?

If you are looking for accelerated results and would like to work with me, the easiest way to do so would be to email me at:

chris@influentialhealthsolutions.com

Please put "Back Pain Solutions" in the subject line, then tell me your name and give me a brief description of what has been bothering you and for how long. I tell people that the time it would take you to heal yourself is 4x greater than if you were working with me. Everybody needs a coach if they want to get to the next level and I'd love to be yours. I look forward to hearing from you if you feel we are a good fit for each other. And don't forget, you can get access to the video course by sending me a simple email. Be happy, be healthy, and be well –

CK

Acknowledgments

My first thank you has to go to my friend, and—although he won't believe it—mentor, Micah Nathan. You sat a cocky, wide-eyed youngster down one day and told me what I needed to do in order to succeed in this business. All roads split out from there and I am where I am today because of that direction. Next, I would like to thank my first and only real boss, Tommy Heffernan. You took a huge chance on bringing me to Hawai'i from Buffalo, New York, gave me way more opportunities than I deserved, fought for me when I messed up, and taught me what it means to live life with a servant's heart. The work you do at the University goes heavily underappreciated in my eyes by those whom you help. Just know I appreciate everything you have done, everything you do, and everything you will continue to do not only for me, but everyone else.

A huge thanks to my younger brother Nick who introduced me to Brian "The Muscle Whisperer" McPherson. Both of you guys opened my eyes to the incredible world of soft tissue manipulation and without your introduction I would have thought pain is something you just get comfortable living with for the rest of your life. To Davone Bess, you helped me get my start as a true professional and trusted me to fix you whenever you had an ache or pain, even avoiding surgery a couple times in the process. Thank you for believing in me and spreading the word. To everyone who came into my gym CrossFit Kismet, thank you for trusting my funky warm-up process where you roll around with a lacrosse ball under your butt and not thinking I was crazy. In some cases, thank you for trusting me with your other friends, and family members, especially your children.

To anyone I helped that was in pain, realize I learned everything I know by allowing me to work with you. Out of all of the books, DVDs, and articles I have studied, you were by far my greatest teacher.

About The Author

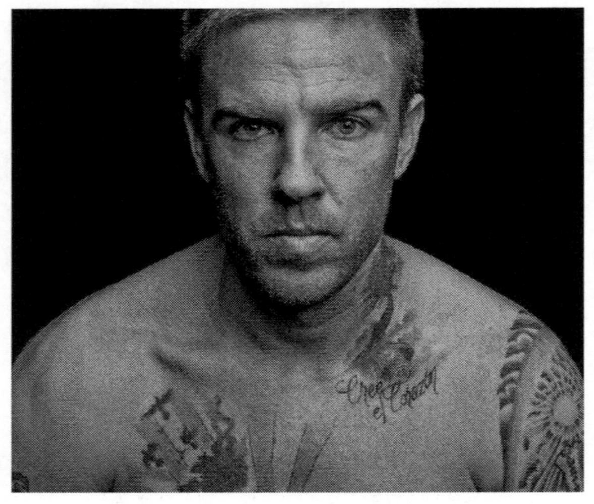

Chris Kidawski has been transforming lives in the health and fitness profession for the last 18 years. Armed with his master's in Kinesiology from the University of Hawai'i, he helps heal and reverse disease from the inside out. Chris has trained people in all walks of life, including but not limited to Navy SEALs, professional athletes, World Champion mixed martial artists, mothers, fathers, sons, daughters, and people just like you!

Chris has dedicated himself to discovering the truth about all aspects of health and wellness and has become as complete of a life coach as you can get. He has written two books so far, *The Death of Dieting*, which teaches you how to detoxify your body with natural, wholesome food, and *The Everspace* which teaches you how to operate from a place of stillness to achieve success in your life.

Chris now lives and runs his business Influential Health Solutions from sunny South Florida, but also does public speaking engagements and seminars in universities and gyms all over the country. He has been featured on many podcasts where he dives deeper into his body/spirit/mind paradigm of human health and thoroughly enjoys opening up people's lives with his information. For speaking inquiries please e-mail Chris at chris@influentialhealthsolutions.com.

You can connect with Chris on his Author Page by going to: https://www.facebook.com/chriskidawski/.

Or on twitter: www.twitter.com/chriskidawski

Lastly, as a self-published author, reviews are worth 10x their weight in gold. If this book touched you in any way, an honest review on Amazon would be extremely appreciated.

You're Giving Back!

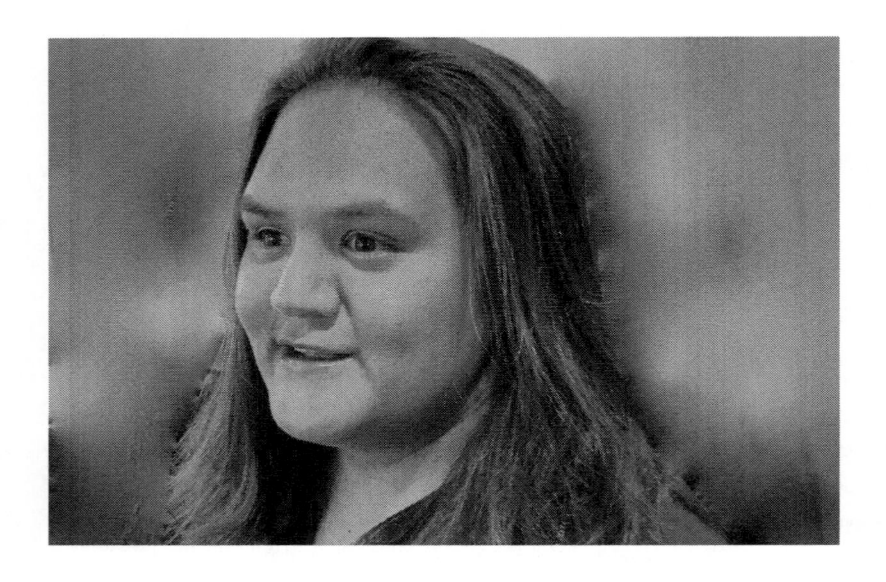

And you don't even know it! Ten percent of the proceeds of my books go to a benefit known as Hilina'i's Walk. Hilina'i is a very special girl who suffers from developmental delays, hypotonia, and emotional outbursts. Throughout her entire life she has fought to overcome many challenges that have come her way. Her condition requires extended individual work with Physical, Occupational, Speech and Psychological Therapists. Our goal is to provide her the opportunity to attend a special needs school that can offer her the services she needs to develop to her full potential. The funds raised from the sales of this book will help to partially cover the expenses for her to attend Variety

School; a school that specializes in special needs children. The school has provided phenomenal results for other children just like Hili unfortunately the cost to send her there is nearly $30,000 per year. If you would like to go above and beyond and make a separate donation, your generosity would be incredibly heartfelt and appreciated by her family. Please send it to:

Hilina'i's Walk
45-212 Makahio St.
Kaneohe, HI 96744

Hilina'i's walk is held every year at the end of July where Hili's father, Tommy, and several other volunteers walk from his home in Hau'ula on the North Shore of Oahu to the school, which is located near Diamondhead crater approximately 37 miles away. Even though volunteers for the walk grow every year, it is getting harder and harder to raise the funds necessary for her education. Mahalo for anything you can give to further this cause.

-CK

Made in the USA
Middletown, DE
18 May 2019